"*What Works When Diets Don't* is a breath of fresh air in the congested market of book publishing. Shane Idleman goes right to the heart of the problem—motivation and information— and helps the reader get back on track. A must-read for anyone serious about health and weight-loss."

– **Dr. Daniel Pompa, author of *Beyond Fasting***

"Shane Idleman knows what it is to be bound, and he knows what it is to be free. He shares the keys to lasting freedom in this practical, inspiring book."

– **Michael L. Brown, Ph.D.,
host of the Line of Fire broadcast**

"Shane has captured the true essence of weight loss! His concise application for getting to the root of weight problems sheds a much-needed new light on taking control over both the physical and spiritual aspects of weight loss."

– **Rodney Corn MA, PES, CSCS,
Director Education, Research & Development,
National Academy of Sports Medicine**

"The wisdom of God's way is always applicable for life, spanning the dimensions from our soul's salvation to our body's health. Shane Idleman is helping us touch the bases wisely —including reaching to touch others with life and grace."

– **Jack W. Hayford, Litt. D.
Pastor/Chancellor, The Church on The Way &
The King's Seminary, Van Nuys, California**

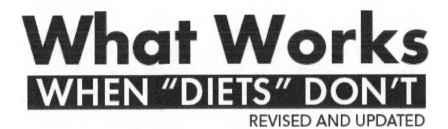

What Works
WHEN "DIETS" DON'T
REVISED AND UPDATED

YOUR PERSONAL 8-STEP
WEIGHT-LOSS SUCCESS GUIDE

SHANE IDLEMAN

El Paseo Publications

What Works When "Diets" Don't:
Your Personal *8-Step* Weight-Loss Success Guide

First edition © 2001 by Shane A. Idleman
Revised edition © 2020 by Shane A. Idleman

Scripture taken from the New King James Version®. Copyright © 1982 by Thomas Nelson. Used by permission. All rights reserved.

Scriptures and quotes within quotation marks are exact quotes; whereas, paraphrased Scriptures and quotes are often italicized.

ISBN: 978-1-7343774-0-8
Published by El Paseo Publications
Printed in the United States of America

Dedication

"When you fall—fall forward!"

This book is dedicated to those who have been discouraged time and time again by repeated efforts to lose weight. My hope is that *What Works When "Diets" Don't* will help you overcome the obstacles that keep you from reaching your goal. It's often said that it's not the fall that hurts but the staying down that does. This book, in addition to helping you lose weight, will encourage you to move forward despite setbacks.

Contents

Disclaimer

This book was written based on personal experience and observation and is sold with that understanding. If professional assistance, other than what is provided, is required, the services of a capable authority are then recommended.

The publisher and the author shall be neither responsible nor liable to any person or entity with respect to damage caused, indirectly or directly, from the information provided in this book. At the time of this writing, free downloads of *Feasting & Fasting* and the author's newest book, *HELP! I'm Addicted*, are both available at WCFAV.org. You can also search Pastor Shane Idleman on YouTube for messages on health, fitness, and fasting.

*Medical note: Before beginning a weight-loss program, it is recommended that you consult your doctor for a checkup because you may place a higher demand on your body than what it has been accustomed to based on your current activity level. If you have any pre-existing problems or health conditions, please see your physician before engaging in any new activities or adjusting food intake.

From the Author

The purpose of this book is to motivate, educate, and encourage success. Although I'm not an advocate of focusing on calories, the adage is true: "If you eat more than your body needs, you will gain weight." Therefore, as a reminder that we must be more active to conquer the obesity epidemic, I do mention caloric intake often.

This book was first published in 2001. It has been republished in 2020 with some minor changes and updates to the original information as well as expanded with the addition of a new chapter. My hope and prayer is that you are encouraged, convicted, and uplifted.

I conclude by thanking my mom, Diane Idleman, for the painstaking process of editing my books over the years. Her suggestions, comments, and edits have made the books what they are today. Thank you, a thousand times over. And a special thank you to my wife, Morgan. We married after this book was released in 2002, and she was very patient during the republishing process that included many edits and updates for the revised edition.

Finally, thank you to Liz Smith at InkSmith Editorial Services. Her insights and suggestions were spot on, as was her editing and publishing assistance. She is a true blessing to any author. Thank you also to Christine Ramsey for taking the time to read through the final manuscript and offer changes the same day I asked—talk about being flexible. And to Susie Woodruff, who manages the church office and allows me the freedom to write when God leads, a heartfelt thank you.

All these people, along with the encouragement I receive from my kids—Aubrey, Shane, Gracie, Kylee, and Madison—made this new release of *What Works When "Diets" Don't* possible. Thank you!

About the Author

Shane Idleman is the founder and lead pastor of Westside Christian Fellowship in Southern California and the author of nine books. His radio program, *Regaining Lost Ground*, can be heard on many different outlets including the WCF Radio Network. More can be found at ShaneIdleman.com, WCFRadio.org, and WCFAV.org.

Pastor Shane began his career in the health and fitness industry in 1992. During this time, he began reading many books and publications from the National Academy of Sports Medicine to better understand how the human body is affected by nutrition and, thus, to equip people with correct information about weight loss.

Shane began compiling this information into an easy-to-read book designed to help others lose weight. After working for nearly a decade with thousands of weight-loss clients in the 1990s, the same questions—as well as the same patterns for success and failure—arose time and time again. *What Works When "Diets" Don't* was developed not only for those who want exact and conclusive answers to their weight-loss questions but also for those lacking the motivation to begin or even restart the process.

Many times, the problem isn't that we raise our standard and miss it, it's that we lower it and hit it.

Introduction

The "D" Word

In times past, the American culture embraced higher standards, such as personal accountability, responsibility, and working toward long-term goals. Parents encouraged their children to work, save, and wait. It's interesting that a less affluent society, then, seemed to produce more in terms of work ethics and an understanding of delayed rewards. With today's focus on instant gratification, however, we often forget how to work toward long-term goals. Yet, I believe we can be just as tenacious and determined today if we focus once again on timeless principles.

Currently, consumers spend billions of dollars—a whopping $72 billion, in fact—each year in the weight loss industry on products such as over-the-counter diet pills, meal replacement shakes and bars, online fitness apps, weight-loss clinics and franchises, and low-calorie frozen meals.[1] Amazingly, in the early 1960s, only 15 percent of adults were on a diet. Now it's been estimated that 45 million of us go on diets each year,[2] and one of the most common New Year's resolutions Americans make is to lose weight.[3]

What's wrong with this picture? These staggering statistics are largely due to the average American's lack of activity and exercise and bad eating habits. Unfortunately, being overweight is not the only problem our sedentary lifestyles and poor diets create, but they can also lead to increased levels of cancer, heart disease, diabetes, strokes, and countless other diseases and illnesses.

It's ironic. We have more fitness centers, personal trainers, and books, journals, and articles written about fitness than ever before, yet health-related illnesses and problems caused by obesity are increasing at an alarming rate. **The state of our society's health will not improve unless we address what we need to hear instead of what we want to hear.**

In general, the word *diet* simply refers to an eating pattern. In the truest sense, we're all on a diet. If your physician were to ask you, "What does your current diet consist of?" they would be asking about your current eating habits. The term *diet* referred to in the title and throughout the pages of this book, however, refers to America's obsession with fad diets and quick weight-loss promises.

I offer thanks to those few in the diet industry whose diet programs focus on health, vitality, education, moderation, sensible eating, and long-term success. To others who are a part of the problem in creating the diet craze, I encourage serious consideration of your responsibility not only to those suffering from obesity now but to the next generation as well.

Eight Steps to Success

In my younger years, I was a manager and a corporate executive in Southern California for the fastest-growing fitness company in the world. Throughout that time, I managed fitness centers and personal training departments while assisting and interviewing thousands of weight-loss clients. As a result, I identified a consistent pattern that surfaced time and time again: Those who were fit rarely, if ever, referred to *dieting*, while people trying to lose weight often referred to being on a "diet." Those who were fit followed a successful weight-loss formula; they didn't diet. As a result of observing this pattern, I've indentified eight steps for successful weight loss, which are outlined in the following chapters.

Eight steps that promote lasting results:

1. Choose to change from the inside out

2. Wisdom: What you don't know *can* hurt you

3. The pain of discipline vs. the pain of regret

4. Prepare to succeed: Setting and achieving realistic goals

5. Make right choices: You make a choice, and it then makes you

6. Prioritize your life: First things first

7. Create lasting change: Maintaining your results

8. The incredible power of fasting

A Different Perspective

Weight-loss books often land at the top of the best-sellers list. As a result, there are several well-written fitness books authored by doctors, nutritionists, and biochemists that discuss, in detail, the weight-loss process. *What Works When Diets Don't* is different. It was written by someone who not only brings the fitness industry perspective but who has personally struggled with weight loss for many years. I reached my weight-loss goal, and you can too! I want to share with you what works, what doesn't, and why. This material will enable readers to reach their goal in the shortest, safest amount of time possible while providing the motivation, encouragement, and support needed to continue.

Motivation is critical to success. Over 60 percent of those who join a gym or begin a diet quit within the first six weeks; their motivation declines because the results they had hoped for are taking longer than planned. *What Works When "Diets" Don't* will help you maintain your motivation during the weight-loss process and beyond. As you begin, it's important to remember that attitude about life's setbacks, and not the setbacks themselves, determine success or failure.

The following chapters will present useful information and success tips while assisting you step by step through the weight-loss process. Your first tip: highlight. Highlight motivational quotes and inspirational stories as you read. Refer to them often. Read and reread. Motivation, like your body, needs constant fuel. Repetition plays a key role in learning. Read and reread while repeating what works.

Throughout my career, it was disheartening to see people set themselves up to fail. Those who "dieted" believed that their short-term effort would produce long-term results. It didn't. Unfortunately, for those interested in quick weight loss, quick weight gain consistently followed. Within the first month, those who diet tend to lose more weight (not necessarily fat) than those who do not diet. After a few months, however, the story is quite different. By this time, the dieter is tired of the restrictive nature and the false expectations that generally accompany dieting. As a result, the dieter resorts to old habits. Weight returns and often increases.

But the person who focuses on long-term success gradually reaches their goal and can change healthy eating patterns in the process. Although he or she may have several ups and downs, they make steady progress. They understand that weight loss is a process. Although it may take some time to reach their goal, they'll be able to enjoy the benefits, hopefully for the rest of their lives.

Enduring Truths

Most of the chapters include a short section at the end entitled "Enduring Truths." These truths have endured the test of time and were designed to promote success, health, and abundant living. Many of man's problems, including health-related problems, could be avoided by simply adhering to these basic principles.

The steps discussed in this book are important for the successful completion of any goal. Although principles such as self-discipline are often considered "higher virtues" that only the "mature" possess, that's clearly not the case. Self-discipline, for example, simply means making a decision to say no (or yes, when appropriate). Learning to apply these well-designed truths can promote success not only in weight loss but in all areas of life. I encourage you not to skip chapters or skim the pages. Each step is a building block to your success and should not be overlooked.

*If I didn't change
my life, my life
would change me.*

CHAPTER ONE

1
Step

Choosing to Change
from the Inside Out

What we *want* to hear
vs. what we *need* to hear

Although I believed I was healthy and fit, by the time I reached my twenty-second birthday, my 6'2" frame had skyrocketed to 270 pounds and I was diagnosed with borderline hypoglycemia. My blood pressure and cholesterol levels were high and my health was rapidly deteriorating. I was told that I might need to take medication for the rest of my life. As a result, I was denied life insurance and was instructed by my physician to "go on a strict diet." I was shocked! I knew that if I didn't change my life, my life would change me!

I immediately drove to a bookstore and purchased a diet book, convinced that it would help. It worked—but only temporarily. Within a few months, I gained back all the weight I had lost. I continued to try different diets for several more years. All of them failed miserably. As a result, I became angry and frustrated. Many of the diets presented *what I wanted to hear and not what I needed to hear* to lose weight and keep it off. It shouldn't be about selling products, pills, and false promises. The truth is that we are losing the war against obesity, and unless we change the way we approach weight loss, it will not improve. Most offer menu plans or diet aids, but the problem goes much deeper and requires more than a quick fix. **We need a solution, not a sales pitch!**

Weight loss is not as difficult as we make it. It becomes more difficult when we waste time on pills and products that don't work. Permanent weight loss and maximum health can only be achieved when the correct information is applied to everyday living and becomes a lifestyle.

You are endowed with the ability to change your life, and it simply begins with a decision. Decide today that you're going to take control and change your life.

Immediate Gratification

With each passing year comes more technical brilliance and unlimited information concerning health and fitness, yet obesity is at an all-time high. Despite the popularity of health and fitness programs, few seem to successfully address our national problem. We cannot continue to be complacent. We, or those we love, have been affected by poor health, mainly due to poor nutrition, obesity, and lack of activity.

I've found that most people want the fastest way to lose weight. But the fastest way is not generally the best way. When we cut corners, results are short-lived. In many cases, "quick" weight loss means starvation and the use of stimulants—and neither produce permanent weight loss. Additionally, there are serious health risks involved. The process of change requires patience, consistency, and obedience in doing what is right.

Unfortunately, we live in an age when immediate gratification has taken precedence over delayed gratification. We are told that weight loss can be quick and easy. As a result, we waste time and money on fitness products that promise the world but fail to deliver worthwhile results. Perhaps you've experienced this before, as have I. There is nothing more frustrating than spending money on weight-loss products that do not work.

A pill may help you lose weight initially because it's an appetite suppressant, but does it keep it off? No, but we want desperately to believe that it can. The majority of diet advertisers thrive on the principle that people will purchase products based on emotional response and urgency. As a result, many have been largely conditioned to believe that they can do the least amount of work possible in the shortest amount of time where weight loss is concerned. That doesn't work, and it never will! **"Lose weight quick" is a great marketing slogan, but it's not realistic.**

An important part of change is changing the way you view the weight-loss process. Set your mind on a slow, consistent pace that will change your habits rather than a "quick fix." The pursuit of immediate gratification, as it relates to weight loss, rarely, if ever, results in success.

Why Don't Diets Work?

Fitness comes with a price, but the dividends far outweigh the ongoing investment. Most people want a general answer that can be applied immediately, but a general answer cannot solve an individual problem.

There is continuing controversy among diet experts concerning what works. One book advises to avoid all carbohydrates, yet another promotes them. Some suggest a high-fat, high-protein diet consisting of no carbohydrates, while others disagree. Who and what do we believe? I'm not discrediting all weight-loss programs and products. Those few who focus on God-given food, permanent lifestyle changes, correct information, and proper supplementation are the most successful.

Most diet books contain some useful information, but many people place all their trust in the book or the diet and not in God, who can change them. As a result, reaching their weight-loss goal becomes impossible because the book was merely an aid—not the solution.

Succeeding at weight loss requires far more than reading a book. It requires the accumulation of knowledge, patience, planning, good choices, support from others, and setting realistic goals. It's been well said that *knowledge is power.*

Diets sell because they give hope and a sense of direction. You may feel that you've finally found the answer to your weight-loss dilemma. But failure is almost always certain because most cannot live with the restrictive or unrealistic nature of today's diets.

Many fail at dieting because they neglect one or more of the eight steps. Good eating habits, for example, are critical to health and fitness, but to rely solely on good eating habits is not necessarily the answer. There are other patterns, in addition to eating correctly, that promote success.

Don't Focus on Dieting

Dieting, as we've come to understand it, causes one to focus more on food, not less! The word *diet* sets the mind for a temporary experience, but a **temporary experience cannot solve a long-term problem.** Failure, then, is programmed before one even begins!

Initially, people are highly motivated and disciplined when they begin a diet. Many immediately stop eating fast food and sweets, quit drinking alcohol, and start exercising excessively. But as time passes, they fail to exercise as often, they don't watch food choices as closely as they once did, and they lose the motivation they previously had. As a result, they fall back into old habits and behaviors.

But you can prevent this happening to you by introducing changes at a *gradual pace.* **What it takes to lose weight is what it takes to keep it off.** Therefore, don't attempt to change your entire lifestyle overnight. For example, cut back on sugar consumption (soft drink, junk food, etc.) and add exercise to your daily routine. A few weeks later, add another day of exercise and limit junk food consumption.

Continue until a balance is reached and you feel in control. If you can cut all the junk food out immediately, more power to you, but be prepared for withdrawals.

Succeeding at weight loss requires a continuous balancing act between choices. If you eat an unhealthy breakfast, for example, you can compensate by eating correctly throughout the rest of the day. Don't get frustrated. The key is to make more right choices than wrong ones.

It's essential to make good choices. Once you make a choice, it then makes you. Choices feed habits, habits define lifestyle, and lifestyle determines your future. Learning to make good choices is an important step in establishing long-term success. You've chosen to change. That change will soon produce new habits that, according to research, can be developed in as little as twenty-one days. Stay with it. **But when you fall—and you will fall—fall forward!** That is crucial to your success. Use the opportunity to learn, and quickly get back on course again. Perseverance leads to success. This principle of perseverance, or falling forward, helped me more than anything else. Don't let discouragement stop you. Move forward! Everyone gets discouraged, but those who learn to move forward despite discouragement eventually reach their destination.

The Right Foundation

In combination, the steps discussed in this book provide the foundation for building a sound weight-loss program. The first step, *choosing to change from the inside out,* is the most crucial but also the most overlooked. **For change to occur on the outside, it must first occur on the inside.** For example, I had to accept my condition of being overweight as a result of the past choices I had made. I stopped blaming people, places, and things and started taking responsibility for my actions, and thus, I took control of my life, asked God for help, and began to move in a positive direction.

If you're blaming circumstances (e.g., genetics, family upbringing), stop! Blame inhibits success. Blame doesn't solve problems—it complicates them. Nor does blame help weight loss—it hinders it. Simply stop blaming and move forward.

Choosing to change your lifestyle from the inside out begins with a choice. *Choosing today changes tomorrow!*

Case in Point: Karen Lacked Confidence

Karen, married and in her mid-thirties, was not able to lose weight despite trying dozens of diets. When I met Karen, she lacked confidence in her ability to succeed. She stated that she had little if any willpower or self-discipline. She couldn't stay motivated. She had been programmed early to fail, carrying messages from the past into the present. Karen was wounded emotionally from a father who consistently pointed out her inadequacies instead of her strengths and from a mother who was indifferent.

Karen's self-image developed early in life and stood in the way of her success. Those most important in her life had never expressed belief in her. In later years, her husband did not realize her need for encouragement. He rarely praised her accomplishments and did little to raise her self-esteem. As a result, she had never accomplished a weight-loss goal.

Karen began to come to the fitness center regularly. Each day I reminded her of her accomplishments thus far and that it was only a matter of time before she would reach her goal. She began to understand how her attitude about herself had hindered her past weight-loss attempts. That was changing! I rallied around what she could accomplish and what she had accomplished.

As the weeks passed, she began to view life differently. She looked forward to each morning with enthusiasm, motivated by reaching one goal at a time. Her new attitude began to affect other areas of her life. Within six months, she achieved her desired weight and felt great. Her accomplishment clearly increased her self-confidence. Her new energy created additional energy. *Her transformation began with a change in attitude from within.*

Karen's story presents a pivotal principle. Negative words as well as a lack of positive words expressed to Karen at an early age played an enormous role in shaping her future. Proverbs states, "Death and life are in the power of the tongue" (18:21). Karen clearly had to overcome a spirit broken through years of ridicule. Select your words mindfully, encourage rather than discourage the success of others, and choose your thoughts carefully in promoting your success.

When it comes to fitness, some people are highly motivated, confident, and fully committed. They count calories, eat healthily, and exercise six days a week. They are dedicated to total fitness. Others are somewhat committed. They desire to lose weight and feel physically fit, but they are not ready to change their lifestyle. And there are those who, like Karen, lack the confidence needed to begin the simplest step of setting a goal. Regardless of motivation level, *the first step is choosing to change.*

Enduring truth: Choosing to change from the inside out

If poor choices have been affecting your health or your overall sense of well-being, simply make a different choice. We were designed to be healthy under most circumstances. Third John 2 states, "Beloved, I pray that you may prosper in all things and be in health, just as your soul prospers." The statement, "as your soul prospers," reminds us that spiritual prosperity is first and foremost; it is fundamental to our overall health and sense of well-being. In short, we can't experience full health and vitality without also considering the health of our soul as our main priority.

While good health should be our goal, there are the unfortunate, unforeseen situations that we do not control. Many of you who are reading this book have tremendous control over the choices you make, but many don't. Be thankful for the control you do have, and let that thought be the catalyst that drives your forward momentum.

Quick Recap: Many times, cultural programming, in the case of poor nutrition, runs contrary to principles that promote good health, and it's important to change the way you think and, thus, choose. Choosing to follow a healthier lifestyle regardless of what today's culture promotes is the first step in reaching your goal.

The Bible has a lot to say about God changing us. When time allows, check out my other books listed at the end of this book. Spiritual health is vastly more important than physical health.

Knowledge plus action equals results. One without the other is like a ship without a course—it's difficult to reach your destination.

CHAPTER TWO

Step **2**

Applying Wisdom—What You Don't Know *Can* Hurt You

O nce you've chosen to change, the next step is to *apply the truth* about losing weight to your weight-loss program. From reading and analyzing dozens of diet books, I noted that, in general, they agree on one fact: success relies heavily on the choices made. While each author encourages the reader to eat certain types of food, not everyone agrees on the same food. Most weight-loss books stop with a discussion of food. However, weight-loss is not only about what we consume but also about education, proper choices, prioritizing, and being prepared.

After years of dieting, I became so frustrated that I almost gave up on fitness altogether. After all, who wants to exercise daily, follow a special diet, and sacrifice time for nothing? We want immediate results. But when the results take longer than what we had planned, we become frustrated and eventually give up. A key element of education is *knowing what to expect.*

Remember, people succeed at weight loss when they stop "dieting" and start focusing on changing their lifestyle. Step outside your comfort zone and be willing to fail. In fact, **successful people fail more than unsuccessful people.** The difference is that successful people don't give up. They get up and move on. Be willing to fail, be willing to learn, and be willing to use both as stepping stones to success. After all, you'll miss 100 percent of the shots you don't take! So stop dieting and start focusing on gradual, healthy lifestyle changes—one day at a time, one choice at a time, one goal at a time.

Case in Point: Randy Was Misinformed

Wisdom, also defined as using good judgment, was lacking for Randy. Randy, a middle-aged male, wanted to lose forty pounds. He used the treadmill faithfully five times a week, but after two months, he had not lost weight. Curious, I asked him how his exercise program was going. He was discouraged because he hadn't lost any weight. I asked about his routine, and he stated that he had heard cardiopulmonary exercise and avoiding fattening foods could help him lose weight. He had only *partial* knowledge. As a result, his diet was extremely high in carbohydrates, supplying over 80 percent of his calories, and very low in fat, supplying 10 percent of his calories. Although the treadmill improved his cardiovascular health, it was not contributing substantially to fat loss because he was consuming more calories than he was burning, and he was eating the wrong type of food.

I recommended he lower his carbohydrate intake to 55 to 60 percent of his daily caloric intake and increase his fat intake. This simple change dropped his overall calorie consumption from over 3,000 to 2,500. We also increased his protein intake to 20–30 percent. Resistance training was immediately added to his program, and we introduced new exercises into his cardiopulmonary routine (e.g., walking up a 5 percent grade on a treadmill for five minutes, followed by a 10 percent grade for five minutes, back down to a 5 percent grade, and repeated for thirty minutes). Within a month, he dropped eight pounds and was well on his way to reaching his goal. Looking back, I would also have suggested intermittent fasting (IF); it works wonders. Back in the 1990s, many of us thought that fasting was bad. We now know better (more about this in chapter 8).

Randy's information was only partially correct. Cardiopulmonary training (cardio) does aid in body fat reduction when used in conjunction with proper eating habits. But fat, although high in calories, should not be eliminated or even minimized most of the time. What we don't know can hurt us and will surely hinder our progress.

Weight Loss: Stick to the Facts

Throughout the years, many incorrect theories have evolved surrounding weight loss. Theories are only that—theories. Stick to facts through proper education. New theories or fads will come and go. There is no simple solution. Hard as the diet industry may try, they'll never reinvent the wheel. The age-old principles discussed in this book have helped many to lose weight. And you can't argue with success. For example, fasting has been around for thousands of years.

Consider the following facts:

➤ The United States consumes more sugar than any other country in the world! Routinely, one American will consume approximately 272 calories a day in added sugar—17 teaspoons each day, which translates to 57 pounds each year![4]

➤ The average American consumes 39.25 gallons of soft drinks each year,[5] or 1,530 grams of sugar (and we wonder why we see record levels of health-related illnesses).

➤ The United States consumes more calories and is less active than a few decades ago. As a result, obesity and obesity-related illnesses are at an all-time high.

➤ One can find thousands of types of diets doing a simple internet search, yet the nation's rate of obesity continues to increase.

➤ The United States reports more health-related illnesses caused by being overweight than any other nation in the world.[6]

➤ The majority of people who diet regain all their lost weight plus more and can even suffer cardiovascular disease, stroke, diabetes and altered immune function by repeatedly losing and gaining weight. Yet lifestyle changes last a lifetime and carry none of the adverse effects of yo-yo dieting.[7]

➤ The CDC reports that two of the four "key lifestyle risks for chronic disease" are poor nutrition and lack of physical activity (tobacco use and excessive alcohol use being the other two), and six in ten adults have a chronic disease.[8]

➤ Our bodies were designed to digest and assimilate God-made food, not man-made food developed in a factory.

➤ Exercise is an important part of a healthy lifestyle. It aids in body-fat reduction and overall cardiopulmonary improvement.

➤ Calories (protein, carbohydrates, and fat) that are not used are stored as adipose (fat) tissue!

➤ Although genes and lifestyle largely influence body composition, both can be successfully addressed.

➤ Carbohydrates, fat, and protein in the correct forms play a key role in the optimal performance and overall health of an individual.

Without question, knowledge concerning long-term weight loss is based on fact, not fiction. If you've read any weight-loss books, you're probably familiar with some of the contradictions:

• Enjoy whatever food you want vs. you can't consume whatever food you want.

• Consume carbohydrates vs. don't consume carbohydrates!

• Eat fat and plenty of it vs. don't eat fat!

• Count calories vs. don't count calories!

• You don't need to exercise to lose weight vs. exercise to lose weight.

The list could go on and on. Who and what should we believe? At this point, many people get discouraged. They have few facts, countless contradictions, and no lasting solutions. And many other facts directly related to health and nutrition are often overlooked. But a key element of wisdom is education.

And what we do know is that sugar, processed food, addiction, and the lack of activity is killing us. The following shocking facts support the importance of proper nutrition and exercise:

1. We refer to being "dangerously overweight" as 20 percent above ideal weight. This can lead to a substantial increase in health-related risks. Obesity has more than tripled since the 1950s.[9]

2. Type 2 diabetes has increased astronomically in the last sixty years. Sadly, it's primarily a lifestyle- and diet-related disease that can be prevented. Diabetes is the leading cause of blindness in people ages 20 to 74,[10] and it ranks number seven on the top ten causes deaths in America. [11]

3. Cancer now affects one in two women and one in three men.[12]

4. Heart disease and cancer take more American lives than any other disease.[13] In many cases, both are related to nutrition.

5. Studies estimate that 1 in 7 cardiovascular deaths are caused by not eating enough fruit, while 1 in 12 are caused by not eating enough vegetables.[14] (It's best to consume most fruits and vegetables raw and organic.)

6. Ninety percent of Americans don't eat enough fruits and vegetables daily. Only 12.2 percent of American adults are meeting the standard for fruit, and 9.3 percent are meeting the standard for vegetables.[15]

7. Smoking, abdominal obesity, high cholesterol, and stress are some of the leading causes of heart attacks. A sedentary lifestyle, diabetes, and eating too few fruits and vegetables also contribute. All of these risk factors are something you control.[16]

Did you know that one piece of bread and a serving of ketchup can contain over a teaspoon of sugar? According to experts, many diseases are preventable through proper nutrition and exercise. Therefore, it behooves us to make a conscientious effort when choosing

the foods we eat, not only for weight management but, more impor-
tantly, for our health. For more information about the role of food in
body composition, see my short book *Feasting and Fasting*.

How Much Is Too Much

Wisdom can be as basic as knowing the recommended serving
size of your favorite foods and choosing correctly. People frequently
ask, *What is a serving size?* Many people simply eat too much food
because they don't recognize the number of calories in a serving size.

And in many cases, the problem isn't eating too much but eating
too often. Choose organic whenever possible. We are what we eat. If
we eat meat, we must choose clean meat and consume it in moderation. I wish we could all farm our own land and milk our own cows,
but that's not realistic for the majority of us. If we eat vegetables and
fruit sprayed with toxic chemicals, they will enter our bodies. For
example, glyphosate, the main ingredient in Roundup weedkill-
er, has been linked to leaky gut, cell damage, and disruption of the
endocrine system, to name just a few damaging effects. Genetically
modified organisms (GMOs) are another hot topic. According to the
Non-GMO Project, "Genetically modified organisms (GMOs) are
living organisms whose genetic material has been artificially manipulated in a laboratory through genetic engineering. This creates
combinations of plant, animal, bacteria, and virus genes that do not
occur in nature or through traditional crossbreeding methods."[17] In
short, if God made it, eat it; if man manipulated it, avoid it. No one is
certain yet of the ramifications of playing God.

Daily Tips

In addition to using wisdom when choosing serving sizes, it's important to acknowledge health studies and incorporate daily tips that
are supported by research. Knowing a few basic nutrition guidelines
can help you make better choices and, thus, increase your knowledge in developing healthy habits.

It's easy to understand why more servings of fruit and vegetables
should be eaten daily. Not only does a serving size contain far fewer calories but the nutritional value alone is also reason enough to

choose from this food group. If you do nothing more than follow this checklist, you'll be well on your way to healthier living:

- Consume **4 to 6 helpings of organic vegetables** daily, preferably at each meal. Generally, 1/2 cup is considered one serving.

- Include **2 to 3 servings of organic fruit** daily. If possible, include a serving at each meal, again, using 1/2 cup serving as your reference. (1/2 cup of strawberries is equal to 25 calories.)

- Consume at least **30 grams of fiber** daily. A pear, for example, contains approximately 5 grams.

- **Fat should come from God-given food** such as flax seeds, olive oil, coconut oil, and avocados. I'm a proponent of eating the actual food versus using the oil. When possible, I use olives instead of olive oil, avocados instead of avocado oil, and almonds instead of almond oil. Not only is the breakdown of the food slower (e.g., low glycemic), the uptake of nutrients and fiber is substantially higher when eating the whole food.

- Depending on your goal (I'm writing to the soccer mom or the average Joe), **protein should be around 15 to 20 percent** of your daily total depending on exercise and activity level (unless your goal is ketosis through a temporary keto eating plan). For example, at 1,500 calories a day, one would consume 75 grams (or 20 percent daily total). Lean meat and fish (not shellfish) are good choices, but I tend to limit meat to 4 ounces a day or every other day or two.

Just as we are permitted to consume meat and dairy, we are also permitted to drink alcohol (although, some of us should abstain)—but we all know about the devastating consequences of overconsumption. Does the same principle of moderation apply to meat and dairy? Granted, meat and dairy advocates such as Weston A. Price have impressive data showing how people have thrived on healthy meat and raw dairy. Some tribes of people eat plant-based food, and others, such as in the Himalayas, eat raw dairy and unprocessed meat; both groups are healthy. The key is that the food is not toxic or sugar-ladened. Ultra-processed foods lead to higher risks of cancer. We reap what we sow. What are you sowing?

- **Water is essential** for health and vitality. Depending on activity and weight, 8 to 12 cups a day is recommended. Choose distilled or clean water whenever possible. Water reduces stress on the heart and aids in overall energy. In addition, protein requires seven times more water for metabolism than carbohydrates and fat.

- **Supplement your meals with a powerful multivitamin and mineral formula.** Choose those that contain high doses of antioxidants and other essential vitamins and minerals. More on this can be found in my book *Feasting and Fasting*.

- **Incorporate intermittent fasting** into your daily routine as well as occasional blocks of fasting. Fasting is a true gift from God with many health benefits. See chapter 8 for more information.

Ingredients: Do You Know What You Eat?

Knowing the ingredients in the foods you consume is crucial to health as well as weight loss. For example, many "diet" products, such as no-calorie sodas and sugar-free ice cream, are artificially sweetened with the controversial ingredient aspartame. When your body processes aspartame, part of it is broken down into methanol. Methanol is toxic in large quantities, yet smaller amounts may also be concerning when combined with some foods.[18]

For decades, I had read that diet soft drinks were not healthy, but that didn't stop me from consuming them regularly. It wasn't until I read *A Consumer's Dictionary of Food Additives* by Ruth Winter that I was convinced and gave up drinking soft drinks for good. These beverages offer zero nutritional value, and their ingredients are harmful.

The heartbreaking truth is that millions of people consume these toxic food additives each day, sometimes several times a day, without realizing what they're absorbing into their bodies. It's little wonder that, as a nation, we're experiencing record levels of health-related problems. Ask yourself, "Does my body need it—or does it want it?" If it needs it, consume it. If it wants it, say no.

I understand that it's not easy to completely quit eating and drinking these products. The media does a masterful job promoting, marketing, and winning our minds with pleasant thoughts associated with their consumption, and we're trained to think that because they are "diet" or "no calorie," it will help us lose weight— in other words, we can have our cake and eat it too. Keep in mind, though, that in most cases profit, not health, drives the food companies!

Many are not concerned about food additives or ingredients because they believe that the FDA offers protection. That's simply not the case. The FDA has admitted that they are no longer an organization focused on prevention but reaction. In other words, the food products in our nation are too numerous for the FDA to regulate; therefore, the majority of the supervision is left to the companies that are producing the products. As a result, the FDA must react to health concerns, not prevent them. You be the judge! Rather than a neutral agency testing without bias, production companies have profit at stake.

Companies are often driven by revenue, and the only one who profits from fasting is the faster. Processed food is cheap and convenient. It often contains stimulating and addictive ingredients and flavor-enhancing chemicals. Keep in mind that terms such as *organic, natural, GMO free, vegan, no trans-fats*, and others are often used for marketing purposes. For example, many popular brands of chips are switching ingredients around so they can place the word *organic* on their packaging, but the product is far from healthy. There are exceptions, but generally, not all products labeled natural or organic are healthy.

Enduring truth: Wisdom—what you don't know can hurt you

Knowledge can be defined as knowing what to do, and *wisdom* is doing what you know. The book of Proverbs describes wisdom as incredibly important for a successful life. Why is wisdom so important? Proverbs 4:7–8 states, "Wisdom is the principal thing; therefore get wisdom. And in all your getting, get understanding. Exalt her and she will promote you; she will bring you honor, when you embrace her." Wisdom is the application of knowledge.

Many fail at dieting because their attempt is not supported by knowledge and its constant application. Scripture advises us to use moderation, choose wisely, and avoid overeating. We now have the technology and research that support these age-old principles for overall health and fitness.

Knowledge enables, empowers, and protects. Understanding your weight-loss process, being consistent, using moderation, and giving it time while developing the principle of perseverance will surely produce results.

There are few greater feelings than controlling our desires rather than having our desires controlling us.

CHAPTER THREE

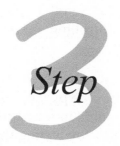

Step

Getting Started—The Pain of *Discipline* or the Pain of *Regret*

Discipline: Is it really important?

s discipline really important? Through extensive contact within
the fitness industry, I found that many people recognized the
need for discipline but believed that they had little if any. They
conditioned themselves to believe that discipline was an attribute
they could not possess. They failed to recognize that they already
possessed it. If it were possible to have offered them a generous sum
of money as soon as they reached their weight-loss goal, they would
have quickly become highly disciplined and lost the desired weight
simply because their motivation outweighed the obstacle. Surpris-
ing, isn't it, because health is far more valuable than money. They
would merely make a choice based on the reward and then act on
that choice—and that, my friends, is discipline.

Discipline is often referred to as training the mind or the body. It's our ability to control our actions and our habits and, thus, our lifestyle. If we exercise discipline in one area, it helps to regulate and strengthen this "control valve" in other areas of our lives. There are few greater feelings than controlling our desires rather than having our desires control us.

When tempted, we should ask ourselves, "Should I pass on this tempting food choice and feel the pain of discipline for approximately five to ten minutes, or should I indulge and experience the pain of regret?" Nothing satisfies like the feeling that you are in control. If you don't control your life, life will control you.

Many authors and diet consultants argue that discipline and willpower cannot change behavior. I agree that discipline alone is not the answer, but totally dismissing it is an invitation for disaster.

Addiction is often referred to as giving oneself up to a habit and then becoming dependent on that habit. Therefore, if the lack of discipline causes bad habits, then the application of discipline, in the right areas, can help produce good habits.

Discipline means staying with whatever it takes to see results. Discipline opens the door to any successful endeavor, while the lack of discipline closes the door. Whether you're building a business, a family, your health, or your education, nothing is built without discipline! Discipline is also an important part of any weight-loss program. Be leery of those who say discipline or willpower isn't important. It's not only important to success—it's essential!

The temporary pain of discipline often leads to fulfillment, pleasure, and overall success. The lasting pain of regret leads to disappointment, discouragement, and frustration. But we can reverse the pain of regret, apply discipline, and experience the great freedom that being in control brings. It's never too late! Are you working hard toward your goals? And are you working smart? Is what you're doing producing the results you want? If not, reconsider what you're doing, and simply make another choice. Replace a poor choice, such as a hot fudge sundae, with a good choice, like strawberries and healthy yogurt. The choice is yours. Again, if you don't control your life, your life will control you. Above all, make the change while you still have the choice.

Discipline is not a mindless, mechanical ritual but rather one that intelligently governs the body by making correct decisions. It can be fueled by the desire to look and feel one's best, or perhaps it is fed by the fear of poor health or an early death. Discipline can be seen as the by-product of motivation. When your discipline fades, revisit the circumstances or goals that originally motivated you. List them again and post them.

Take two steps forward, forget the one step back, and eventually, you will reach your goal. Remember, a temporary step back does not have to be a permanent setback unless you fail to move forward. The ability to properly apply discipline is what separates those who succeed from those who almost succeed.

Many of you reading this book may not feel that you have enough discipline to exercise or eat correctly. Don't worry, neither did I initially. It's simply a process that starts by making better choices. Many of the articles and books I read while trying to lose weight said that willpower and discipline weren't needed to lose weight, but that can be misleading. It wasn't until I incorporated discipline that I started seeing measurable results. I soon realized that discipline is a by-product of motivation. I didn't necessarily lack discipline—I lacked motivation.

Case in Point: Almost Too Late for Chris

Chris, a fifty-four-year-old female, was active in her teens, but an injury in her twenties set her back. She had neglected her health for several years, and this pattern eventually developed into a dangerous lifestyle.

She was diagnosed with high blood pressure, high triglyceride levels, and extremely low HDL levels (good cholesterol). Her doctor warned her that she was a candidate for developing diabetes and other health-related illnesses. At this point, she had a choice: to encounter the pain of discipline in changing her lifestyle or experience the lasting pain of regret, ill health, and possible early death.

The decision was easy. Remarkably, after forty-five days of exercise and proper nutrition, Chris' blood pressure and triglyceride levels dropped significantly, and the HDL count increased.

However, within six months, she was back where she started. Her old habits and lifestyle again claimed her health, and a few years later, she was scheduled for heart surgery. Yet, after surgery, she resumed her exercise and healthy eating routine, this time for good. Her failing health had motivated her to begin, and as a result, her discipline increased. Again, she didn't lack discipline—she lacked motivation.

I know of countless others who have avoided surgery by changing their lifestyle and their diet. But why do we wait? Why do you wait? Unfortunately, it took an extreme circumstance to get Chris back on track. Don't make the same mistake. Make a decision to change today and avoid the pain of regret tomorrow.

Focus on Strengths and Identify Weaknesses

It's important to identify both strengths and weaknesses before starting a weight-loss program. An assessment of your traits may reveal addictions or dependencies. For this book, an addiction is defined as any repeated behavior that negatively affects your health, your family, or other important areas of your life. Addictions are not easily addressed because patterns are often deeply rooted. Addictions that are responsible for weight gain must be addressed for weight loss to occur.

Overuse of or dependencies on food, alcohol, or certain drugs make it very difficult to lose weight. For example, I have spoken with literally thousands of people who temporarily gave up drinking alcohol to lose weight or to redeem a broken relationship. But because the addictive nature was not addressed, it eventually surfaced again. They made a temporary commitment believing it would end a long-term problem. A commitment to change must be a lifelong commitment, which includes losing weight.

Another important step, although extremely difficult, involves removing addictive substances that undermine health. I vividly remember a comment from a clinical nutritionist that motivated me: "Discontinuing caffeine intake leads to significant improvements in health, far more than just dieting alone." He also made the connection between depression, anxiety, and panic attacks to excessive caffeine.

Don't get me wrong. As a person who once loved a few strong cups of coffee, I understand that moderation is the key. But when the body is kept in a constant state of stress, no wonder it breaks down often and why many never overcome fatigue. Contrary to popular belief, stimulants don't help fatigue; they contribute to it by robbing Peter to pay Paul.

Since caffeine runs along the same biochemical pathways in the brain as cocaine, opium, and amphetamines, quitting can be a nightmare. My suggestion is to back off day by day until intake is very minimal and use organic green tea (light caffeine) whenever possible. You'll be shocked by the results. Granted, the first week to ten days may be torture, but it will be worth it. The withdrawal symptoms alone reveal the power of this drug. I was fascinated to read that the logo of a very popular coffee franchise represents a seductive image that allures and entices. How ironic.

The *Diagnostic and Statistical Manual for Mental Disorders* now recognizes caffeine-related disorders such as caffeine intoxication, caffeine-induced anxiety disorder, and caffeine-induced sleep disorder. These can begin with even minimal doses. Increase the amount to 500 mg of caffeine (the amount found in approximately 24 ounces of coffee), and these symptoms are dramatically increased. All this can lead to angry outbursts, panic attacks, severe depression, and extreme irritability. This begs the question, How many are suffering mentally and physically simply because of poor health—continuing the addiction rather than removing the cause of the problem? Not in all cases but in most, depression, anxiety, irritability, and so on could be severely curtailed if health (spiritual and physical) was a priority.

In the same way that a hiker feels released, energized, and unburdened after removing a fifty-pound backpack, you'll feel released and energized after removing stimulants. I became kinder and more patient and easygoing after I quit abusing coffee. I never realized how much it was contributing to my anger, irritability, mood swings, and anxiety until at least a week after weaning off, and the withdrawals brought out the worst in me. I always excused my poor attitude with statements like, "I had a bad day," "I'm under a lot of stress," or "I'm tired." Ironically, *I* was the primary cause of my bad days, stress, and fatigue. As much as I wanted to be filled with the Spirit, I was feeding my body a substance that was counterproductive.

Remember, your main goal is health, and stimulants aren't healthy. Ask yourself, *What is the risk to my health versus the benefit to my health?* Will the benefits outweigh the risks? No. Your heart and organs work very hard, and they don't need the added stress.

Consider again two important choices of planning for success: discipline and regret. One produces change, the other hinders it—unless you learn from it. Do what it takes to make the necessary changes in your life to offset the addictive behavior, and your odds of success will greatly increase.

As you begin, identifying those things early that might underscore your success will help you prepare for them in advance. On the other hand, as you identify your strengths, you can actively utilize them to obtain success. Focus on your strengths throughout your weight-loss program.

Identify strengths and weaknesses

Example:

Weakness: I'm not disciplined when it comes to exercise

Strength: I'm good at reaching any goal I set and staying committed

In this example, the person would set a realistic exercise goal that would support commitment. Instead of trying to exercise six days a week, they would begin by exercising twice a week. As their level of discipline increases, they would add an extra day of exercise to their program.

Although the following exercise is basic, it will help you formulate a plan. *Without a plan, there is no direction, and without direction you'll miss your goal.* Remember, if you don't know where you're going, you'll probably get there.

Take time and list three major obstacles (weaknesses):

Example: *Binge eating in the evenings*

Then list three ways to overcome or offset them. Binging is often the result of starving the body throughout the day. To offset binging, try to consume ample amounts of nutrient-dense food throughout the day (e.g., fruits, vegetables).

Identifying your strengths and primary weaknesses can help offset potential problems. If you're having a difficult time identifying your strengths and weaknesses, remember that your strengths can be seen in what you stand for, your weaknesses in what you fall for! In other words, your strengths are strong character traits that allow you to make the right choices; your weaknesses are areas in character that cause you to make wrong choices (e.g., lack of commitment, lack of patience) Be on the lookout, and avoid situations that may cause you to fall. Change your position while you're still in control.

Forget the Past, Possess the Future

Research has found that those who succeed are those who continue through delays. Forget past failures to lose weight. Instead, decide what you're going to do with the days, weeks, months, and years ahead. Plan your time, or your time will plan you. Don't live with ongoing regret. Take control of your life and change your direction. Don't look back unless it's the direction you want to go. You can't change where you've been, but you can change where you're going. The apostle Paul said it best: "But one thing I do, forgetting those things which are behind and reaching forward to those things which are ahead" (Philippians 3:13).

The first step you take toward your goal soon becomes the second, the third, and the fourth. Diligently, step by step, you've reached your goal, and *yesterday's goal becomes today's reward.*

You possess tremendous inner power and strength. You've been given the power to make decisions, the power to develop habits, and the power to choose at any given time. Position yourself to succeed, and choose the momentary pain of self-discipline rather than the nagging pain of regret.

Enduring truth: The pain of discipline or the pain of regret

Discipline, also known as *self-restraint, self-control,* or *obedience,* is an enduring truth that undergirds any successful endeavor, including weight loss. Many are willing to break a habit, lose weight, improve a marriage, attend church, or seek God more fervently, but willingness alone is not enough. Willingness must be followed by action, and action is the result of discipline.

It is important to exercise control when you are still in control or at your greatest level of control. Once things get out of hand, it's more difficult to stop the momentum. Say no before the challenge becomes too great. When things do get beyond you, remember you'll have another opportunity to avoid them next time.

A structure is only as strong as its foundation. Therefore, step by step, the foundation of a successful weight-loss program is being developed. The foundation of your program (e.g., the eight steps) is crucial because everything that follows depends on the integrity of that foundation. Your success is directly related to the strength of the foundation. If it's strong, progress is more easily achieved. If it's weak, success becomes very difficult.

As we move into step four, let's revisit the first three steps.

1. Commit yourself to a lifestyle change. Change your perception of weight loss, and prepare for steady success, not quick fixes (choosing to change from the inside out).

2. Know the facts about nutrition and weight loss while constantly applying education to your weight-loss program (what we don't know can hurt us).

3. Choose discipline over regret. Take control early while you're still in control.

Stay focused on the goal, not the challenges.

CHAPTER FOUR

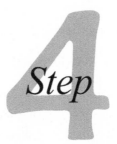

Step

Preparation—Setting and Achieving Realistic Goals

Preparing for Long-Term Success

When establishing a goal, it is crucial to plan for the future and prepare for the present. You've made the choice to change, acquired a better understanding of how your body works, and are learning to choose self-discipline over regret. Now design a plan.

Having a plan is essential, *but it's of no importance if you're not prepared.* Prepared for what? Prepared for unforeseen circumstances, illness or injury, and the challenging but rewarding opportunities ahead.

Many who lose interest in exercising and eating correctly do so because they are not prepared for the interruptions and distractions that can break the routine. How many times has sickness or a vacation derailed our goals? A successful weight-loss program will encourage you to continue, regardless of your situation. People fail at weight loss not because they're defeated but because they quit. Those who succeed are those who continue despite delays.

Case in Point: Lisa Was Discouraged

Lisa, a thirty-eight-year-old mother of two, wanted to lose twenty pounds in three months. She had a plan: Work out six times a week, one hour each time, and consume 1,400 healthy calories a day. Theoretically, this could work, but **life happens.** Within the first three weeks one child became ill, and her car needed repairs. Frustrated and off course, she consumed more than her body needed and was only able to exercise a little. As a result, she lost two pounds within the first month instead of the expected six or seven.

The second month brought even more challenges. The babysitter canceled twice, and Lisa had to attend school functions, work longer hours, and sacrifice her time for friends in need. As a result, she lost two additional pounds instead of the six she had hoped for. She didn't make it to the third month. Discouraged, she quit. She was not prepared for unforeseen circumstances. Instead of focusing on the weight that was lost and improved health, she focused on her failure and quit. A simple readjustment in her goal and attitude would have brought success, but we often look for excuses to continue in a harmful lifestyle. Excuses must end.

By gradually losing the weight, Lisa could have still reached her goal. In allowing more time, she would have encouraged the development of new, enduring patterns. Being prepared and setting realistic goals would have probably meant Lisa's success.

I'm not a fan of always monitoring calories because it can become a form of dieting, but it is important that people know what they are consuming, at least initially. For example, many people trying to lose weight drink a lot of juice because it's healthy. Yes, homemade juice does have benefits, but it's also high in sugar, and it contains approximately 120 calories per cup. That adds up.

Be prepared for setbacks, and continue despite being set back. I have setbacks every week, but my focus is on the end of the race, not the falls here and there. In Lisa's case, she could have still eaten very clean and incorporated intermittent fasting, which would have given her energy and weight loss. Physical and mental preparation promotes success. Again, the best preparation is to decide that you'll move forward regardless of your situation. Be prepared for a slow but steady pace.

Weight loss is a gradual process. Many give up simply because they are not prepared for the time it takes to lose weight.

If you have a financial setback and can't afford healthy food, you can still eat God-given food and apply intermittent fasting to your daily schedule. If you're sick, consider fasting or sipping bone broth, not ice cream and pastries. If you're on vacation, choose to be selective. I look forward to our vacations. I bring plenty of healthy food, exercise by hiking and walking, and enjoy a treat now and then. Last year I came back from vacation four pounds lighter.

Prepare yourself mentally as well. For example, it may take four, six, eight, twelve, or more months to lose forty, sixty, or a hundred pounds or more (depending on your food choices and activity level). Set a goal to lose three to five pounds the first month, and focus on nothing but reaching that goal. The following month, focus on losing three to four more pounds, then three to four more, three to four again, and so on while adjusting when needed. Breaking a large goal into smaller goals can make each easier to reach, with the same amount of enthusiasm and intensity as the first goal. But don't focus on weight loss—instead, focus on health.

Many who focus on weight loss only cut corners and compromise their health with stimulants and weird diets. Even if you maintain your weight for a week or two, don't get frustrated. The body is cleansing at the cellular level, and that can take time, or you may need to break the plateau cycle. Only weigh yourself once a week with the same scale at the same time each day. I encourage measurements over monitoring weight (or both). Muscle is dense and affects body weight; measurements give a better gauge overall.

For my weight-loss goal, I took my time, exercised moderately, ate correctly 80 percent of the time, expected setbacks, and planned mentally as well as practically. For example, I wanted to lose my weight in four months, but as the months went by, I realized that it might take an additional month or two. As a few more months passed, I realized it might take even longer. But eventually, I reached my goal. I didn't starve myself, go on a "diet," or always work out twice a day. I made realistic changes and approached life day by day, adjusting my goals accordingly.

The extended time it took to reach my goal helped me to develop more deeply ingrained habits and an appreciation for perseverance and commitment. I focused on the rewards of weight loss, not the weight-loss process. It's truly that simple, but because we want quick results, we cut corners and sabotage our weight-loss progress.

Ironically, when we choose God-given, healthy food (not processed, boxed, or altered), the body is more apt to lose weight. For example, if you're eating sugar throughout the day, guess what your body will crave? Sugar! Many times, when I avoid food all day and eat a large, healthy dinner between 5 and 7 p.m., I have no sugar cravings nor do I wake up late at night craving more food.

If you fall short, adjust your goal and move forward. Fall forward.

Motivation by Association

Without a doubt, maintaining motivation is a major challenge and requires focused attention, but there's plenty of help.

In my twenties, with pending health problems, the decision was easy. I wanted to live a healthy, productive life. Once I made that choice, my actions reflected that decision. I didn't always make the right choices, but my commitment was strong enough to keep me on track, and I learned to make more right choices than wrong ones.

Our actions in life determine our outcome in life. Motivation is the by-product of a determined commitment to live a healthier life, lose weight, and so on. Long-term goals drive long-term motivation. Many do not think long-term; they generally set two- or three-month weight-loss goals so they can go back to junk food when the diet is over. Remember, health is a lifelong goal.

Motivation is short-lived when commitment is short-lived. Motivation is fueled by momentum, and like the body, it must be fed often. Surround yourself with those who press, not depress, you. It's a fact that those you associate with as well as your surroundings greatly influence you. Whenever possible, associate with people who will encourage you to raise your standard and keep it there. Again, many times the problem isn't that we raise our standard and miss it; it's that we lower it and hit it!

I often meet with people who share similar goals and interests. By association, I'm highly motivated. The Bible, for example, refers to being equally yoked. The primary context of the verse refers to marriage, but the principle is that companions, good or bad, influence character.

We can't deny the timeless principle of fellowship as it relates to motivation and encouragement. For that reason, I encourage you to become involved in a group that will meet regularly to encourage success, not only in weight loss but in all areas of life.

Motivation by association also includes the media. I am constantly encouraged through motivational teachings and radio programs. (Check out WCFRadio.org for added motivation and spiritual encouragement.) It's especially important to stay motivated through the most difficult times. However, much of today's media is not motivating but, rather, "de-motivating." Therefore, spend your time wisely and listen only to those programs that motivate you to succeed and strengthen your relationship with God. I started a YouTube page for this very reason— to motivate and educate.

Motivation means the same as *incentive, enthusiasm, impulse, driving force, and purpose,* and all promote the completion of a successful weight-loss program. Find what drives you, and then drive hard! How about energy to enjoy life with your kids or grandkids? How about being healthy so you can do more for God and others? How about influencing others around you? The obesity rate for kids is alarming. Parents who pack the pantry and load the refrigerator with junk food need to reevaluate what they are doing

Are You Pulling Over or Driving?

Many people pull over more than they drive. Or they take detours, experience delays, and hit roadblocks, and that's it—they quit! My detours were negative relationships I exchanged for those that drove me to higher standards. Experiencing delays represented making wrong choices. Again, I eventually learned to focus on making more right choices than wrong ones. Roadblocks are unforeseen obstacles. Don't let them hold you back—find a way around or through, and move forward again.

Discover what motivates you, and keep feeding that passion. I've discovered that purpose, positive passion, and motivation go hand in hand. Motivation is fed by passion, and passion, by purpose. Prayer and constant focus on the Word of God have been the greatest contributing factors in maintaining my motivation and personal fulfillment, not only in physical health but in spiritual health as well.

Making the right choices encourages motivation. Even during difficult times, spiritual strength and the added boost of physical health produce a better state rather than a bitter state.

We are encouraged to stay motivated and to fight the good fight, but because many are not looking to the right source for their motivation, they never find it. From my experience, God blesses discipline, rewards perseverance, and honors commitment.

Moving Away from the Harbor

From time to time, you may feel helpless and depressed while trying to lose weight because weight loss is taking longer than planned. You may even lose confidence in your ability and feel like giving up and returning to your familiar comfort zone. DON'T! This thinking is absolutely wrong! Press through. You are developing the important principle of perseverance.

There is a saying that "ships are safest in the harbor, but they are not made for the harbor." Likewise, God designed you to weather the storms of life. When life becomes difficult and challenging, set your sights on your goal, not the challenge, and pass through.

As a Christian, you were not created to fail—you were created to succeed. There may be a blessing just beyond the circumstance, or God may be deepening your relationship with Him. Simply trust God despite appearances, and keep moving forward.

Yes, life can be difficult and challenging, but that shouldn't be a reason to give up. Instead, it should be a reason to fight back. How you *respond* to a situation is just as important and, in many cases, more important than the situation itself.

When you allow your emotions to dictate your actions, you lose control of the situation. Being overweight may be your present circumstance, but it does not have to be your future condition. Remember, you were created to weather the storms successfully. Apply what it takes to stay your course. Many are somewhat prepared for the physical exertion it takes to lose weight, but few prepare for the mental exertion. Use the calmer times of your life to prepare for the challenges ahead, not only physically but also mentally. Much like an athlete who prepares physically and mentally all year for the one-day event, he or she doesn't win the event in one day; it is a gradual practice of preparation, discipline, and perseverance. Small victories earned day by day produce winning results. We play like we practice: prepare in the harbor but be ready for the turbulent sea.

Remember, motivation is fueled by success. Little successes day by day will keep the fire of motivation going. Motivation is the drive inside all of us that causes us to act. Without it, we wouldn't get out of bed in the morning. Maintaining your motivation lies within your ability to wait for delayed gratification and to set realistic goals. Remain focused on your goal and not on your current situation. Your hard work will pay off. It's not a matter of if but when.

Motivation and goal setting share a circular relationship: motivation moves us toward our goal, while reaching our goal fuels our motivation. Stay focused. Motivation is a key ingredient to a successful weight-loss program.

Quick, Simple, and Easy Weight Loss

In general, the diet industry as well as the media promote weight loss as being simple and easy, that it only takes a few minutes a day to see results if you take or use this or that product. They have programmed the consumer with preconceived ideas about losing weight that are absolutely false. It's no wonder that people are having a difficult time losing weight; they're not prepared for what lies beyond the pill, product, or thirty-day diet. False information has programmed an attitude doomed to fail.

Think about this for a moment. What if you had been conditioned to believe that after you turned eighteen all your challenges would be over—that money grew on trees, you'd be able to slide right through life without any problems, and people would always treat you with respect? Can you imagine the shock and dismay you would experience when none of that came true? The same is true of weight loss. What the diet industry tells society, society will believe as truth.

Did you ever really find that miraculous product that promised to change your life? Neither did I, but we all want solutions to our weight-loss problems, and we're willing to pay large sums of money in pursuit of the answers. Many businesses know this, and they make a profit by selling false hope.

I recently saw an advertisement on television promoting a small piece of home-exercise equipment as capable of great things. I do believe that home exercise equipment can help, but claims such as "It only takes a few minutes a day" and "You can eat whatever you want" can be misleading. They're not giving the consumer all the information they need to lose weight effectively. In fact, they're adding to the rising level of obesity by providing false expectations about weight loss. To add fuel to the fire, the actors in the commercial were in phenomenal shape, contributing their success to the equipment and not an overall lifestyle. We shouldn't be surprised. Companies that are production driven without being character driven often focus on the wrong goal!

But what if the diet industry took a different approach? What if they educated people about fitness and gave us the tools we need to succeed such as support, encouragement, and direction? What if they instead said, "It may not be easy, but it will be the best change you've made. Let us show you how." Can you imagine the difference that would make? That's exactly what I'm trying to convey in this book. I want to teach you how to succeed on your own without pills, products, or false promises. I want to prepare you for the process.

Being prepared for the weight-loss process allows you to overcome obstacles, not be caught off guard and overwhelmed by them. Fortunately, most fitness centers often encourage ongoing commitment and motivation and offer the assistance of personal trainers for continuous support.

And when we are persistent and committed, when we do not give up, and we continue to press toward the goal despite obstacles, we approach life more successfully. Thus, we are prepared for the future, not surprised by it.

Society's Influence

We can't purchase weight loss. We have to acquire it through action and effort. In most cases, the quicker you lose weight, the more difficult it is to keep it off. Many products and pills promise quick results but rarely deliver.

Be prepared by asking two questions. First, is what the product claiming to do realistic? It's not possible to see your abdominal muscles in two short weeks if you have a lot of weight to lose. Use common sense, and think before you buy. Home exercise equipment, for example, may aid in body fat reduction, but without incorporating lifestyle changes, it will not, in itself, be the answer. Second, is the product (e.g., pills) safe? What are the effects that it will have on the body (e.g., rapid heart rate, elevated blood pressure, mood swings)? If it's not realistic, safe, or healthy, don't use it.

We tend to rush the weight-loss process because society has placed a high premium on outer appearance and instant gratification. Many people spend most of their lives trying to look different or like someone else. They rate their appearance by society's standard. They search for fulfillment, striving to look like the perfect "10." Unfortunately, this false perception causes many people— even the 10s—to remain unfulfilled! When we compare ourselves to one another, we are just not being wise. You weren't designed to be someone else; you were masterfully designed to be you. If you're trying to be someone else, you may miss God's plan for *your* life.

A perfect physique does not guarantee happiness any more than a good mattress guarantees sleep. True happiness does not come from outer appearance but from knowing God. However, physical fitness can help. Spiritual, physical, and emotional health can add years and quality to life. Together they maximize your greatest potential. Physical fitness can help strengthen all areas of your life. It provides you with the energy to deal with life's challenges, the strength to press through, and the ability to continue regardless of your circumstance. Certainly, some people do not possess physical health but are spiritual giants, and I greatly admire them. This message is intended for those have the ability to increase their physical health.

Life pushes and pulls, and it will draw you into battles you are ill prepared to withstand unless you are fit physically and spiritually. Physical fitness, like spiritual fitness, can aid in the development of discipline, strength, patience, confidence, endurance, and commitment. These qualities are fundamental to success in life as well as in weight loss.

Focus on the end result of your hard work. Placing your emphasis on the goal, not the challenge, makes it easier to persevere. Stop aiming for quick, simple, and easy, and start focusing on lasting, worthwhile results.

Be Prepared: Helpful Tips

1. Since the cost of healthy food can get expensive, trying looking for sales at a few different stores. I often find organic eggs at 50 percent off if they are near the expiration date. Boil them, and they'll last another week. Buy organic fruits and vegetables as much as possible, but definitely when purchasing any of the "Dirty Dozen" (strawberries, kale, spinach, etc.), which are heavily sprayed with chemicals.[19] If your budget is tight, buy nonorganic varieties of the "Clean Fifteen,"[20] use only one scoop of healthy protein powder instead of two, and take supplements

three times a week rather than every day. Instead of asking, "Why is good food expensive?" we should ask, "Why is bad food so cheap?"

2. Reallocate your money. Many people spend at least $10 a day at their favorite coffee house. That can add up to $300 a month. Use that money instead to purchase healthy food.

3. When you begin to exercise, expect to hit a wall within the first five or ten minutes. You may feel like quitting, but don't. Many times, your energy level will dramatically improve within a few minutes, and you'll finish your workout with energy to spare.

4. The busier you stay throughout the day (e.g., working, cleaning, running errands, hobbies), the less likely you'll be to snack or splurge. The solution: move more, sit less! Immediately following a meal, stay busy—somewhere other than the kitchen, if possible. Allowing yourself to think about additional food will only fuel your appetite. You may even believe that you're still hungry.

5. Incorporate intermittent fasting and long fasting (more in chapter 8).

6. Avoid diet drinks. Diet drinks and other products that contain artificial sweeteners can often dehydrate and eventually sap energy—and that's only a few of the health risks associated with their consumption. Eliminating these products can increase long-term energy and decrease overall appetite.

7. If you're going to exercise mid-afternoon or evening, some experts suggest that it's often best to perform resistance training before cardiopulmonary training (e.g., thirty minutes of weights followed by thirty minutes of jogging, power walking, or biking). This allows for a substantial portion of your glycogen storage (energy) to be used during the resistance training phase of your program, thus causing your fat storage to be used as the *primary* fuel during the cardiopulmonary training phase.

8. If your plan is to exercise first thing in the morning, some suggest consuming a small amount of protein beforehand, such as a protein shake. This helps to minimize muscle tissue from being

broken down and converted to fuel and provides the needed energy. However, others advocate exercising on an empty stomach. Working out during a fast of 12 to 18 hours can be beneficial. If cardiopulmonary training is done upon awakening on an empty stomach, fat storage is more readily available for fuel. While muscle can also be used as fuel during this type of energy expenditure, God designed us to go into "protein sparing" mode where our body spares muscle and burns fat (ketones). Therefore, I prefer not eating before exercising.

9. If, within an hour or two after eating, you feel hungry again, persevere through it. The supposed "hunger" eventually leaves. We really aren't hungry during these times of cravings. Our bodies have been conditioned over the years to eat more than we need.

10. Plan daily meals whenever possible. *Pre-planned means prepared.* Knowing ahead what to eat and having it available will help avoid reaching for just anything when hungry. Before leaving for work in the mornings, I'd often fill my cooler with tuna or sodium-free turkey sandwiches, low-fat cottage cheese, delicious oat bran bars, grapes, apples, pears, and vegetables. This allowed me to stay within my daily caloric allowance and consume only healthy foods. In addition, my food was already prepared for the day, and I wasn't forced to resort to fast food to satisfy my hunger. This is truly the *fastest* fast-food approach.

11. If you fail to eat properly for a day or two in a row, don't worry. Start the following day with a new, forward-moving attitude. Check your refrigerator and cupboards; do you need to add or subtract? Within a few weeks, expect to repeat the process again. The key is to begin to make more right choices than wrong ones.

12. Read reputable health and fitness magazines often enough to keep your education and motivation on track.

13. When possible, walk, jog, or hike outside. Fifteen to twenty minutes in one direction gives no other choice than to continue fifteen to twenty minutes in the other direction. Fitness facilities are great for resistance training (weight training) because they

offer many types of equipment as well as the availability of personal trainers.

14. When exercising, choose audio (or video) messages that motivate and increase your knowledge. I often listen to business briefings, sermons, and other educational material when exercising. This increases my motivation to exercise. I look forward to the opportunity to increase my knowledge and to exercise at the same time.

15. Don't allow yourself to fall into the "winter weight-gain trap" that starts in October and ends in January. Many use the winter months as an excuse to gain weight—sometimes twenty pounds or more! Stay focused, and stay on top. Never gain more than a few pounds throughout the winter season. Again, a successful weight-loss program focuses on lifestyle changes, not temporary changes. Conceding in the winter and trying to regain lost ground in the spring and summer is not a productive lifestyle. Enjoy and embrace the holidays, but focus on moderation.

16. Avoid buying food that you'll be tempted to eat. For example, I rid my home of unhealthy treats, breakfast cereals loaded with sugar, chips, and other tempting foods. I found that the best solution for me was *out of sight, out of mind*. In time, you'll lose much of your desire for these foods.

17. Schedule exercise with other important daily activities. Prioritize—put first things first!

18. Although many diet books and magazine articles contain helpful information about weight loss, they are not the answer in themselves. Neither is home exercise equipment. These may help you to lose weight initially, but it's persistence, correct information, and moving forward despite setbacks and circumstances that are your most valuable tools in losing long-term weight and staying fit. They will catapult you toward your success.

19. Use wisdom. Do not believe claims such as "it only takes a few minutes a day" or "you can consume whatever you want, just take this pill before or after eating" or "lose all the weight you want while you sleep." These claims develop a false perception

about weight loss for consumers. Again, use common sense. If it sounds too good to be true, it probably is!

Important Note: Not all calories are the same. Just look at wild animals; we don't see too many that are overweight unless they are fed processed food. For example, 120 calories of nuts are better absorbed and utilized than 120 calories coming from a candy bar. Not only is less insulin released, but your body will also utilize more nutrients, thus reducing cravings. And fiber from the nuts will be used to carry food waste out of your system, something a candy bar has a hard time doing. Eating less and moving more is not always the solution. A slow metabolism, hormonal imbalance, or thyroid issues can also play a role. If you simply eat less, your metabolism may slow even more. The key is to eat God-given foods in their purest form while exercising more often.

The First Four Building Blocks of Success

The first four steps—choosing to change from the inside out, educating yourself, choosing discipline over regret, and preparing for the setbacks—all promote long-term success. You've made the decision to change your life. You are increasing your knowledge concerning healthy eating habits, and you have given thought to the pain of discipline and the pain of regret. You're now better prepared for the weight-loss process. Move forward to step five: making the right choices. Again, we're building a foundation. The stronger the foundation, the better to weather the storms!

Enduring truth: Preparing for long-term success

Wisdom, as well as history, tells us that we cannot defeat an enemy we cannot see. Furthermore, we surely cannot win if we're not prepared.

Two types of preparation can aid in our success: *practical* and *mental* preparation. Practical preparation includes shopping ahead, setting realistic goals, being prepared for "off days" and those triple-calorie meals, and at times, days of interruptions. However, the most important preparation is mental and spiritual preparation. Challenges are merely opportunities to develop spiritual muscle. Being prepared, overcoming the hurdles, and keeping your course will help you reach your goal. Don't give up. Know that challenges are only temporary step-backs and not permanent setbacks!

Preplanned Means Prepared

How are you preparing? List your goals and refer to them often. This will help you stay on track. Take a few minutes and state what you want to accomplish. Remember, if you don't know where you're going, you'll probably get there.

The following tips are those that others have used to successfully change habits. This is just a start to your checklist to success; add other tips as you learn them through the process:

__ Begin preparing your body for fasting by missing a meal or two and consuming nothing but clean water.

__ Rid your home of any food that will hinder progress.

__ Enroll in a health club or begin walking and exercising at home. You don't need a fancy workout plan. Simple sit-ups, squats, and presses do wonders. Turn off the television and begin moving.

__ Set realistic time frames to accomplish your goals.

__ List your favorite healthy foods, and shop primarily from this list.

__ Enlist a friend to exercise with you or begin to exercise on your own—exercise accelerates weight loss.

__ Use a central area to keep inspiration and education in focus. A bulletin board works very well.

Top Five Common Obstacles and Their Solutions

Obstacle: Caving in when tempted

Solution: Out of sight, out of mind; don't have tempting foods nearby.

Obstacle: Discouragement

Solution: Success doesn't come without failure. Get back on track, and learn from the experience. Don't give up.

Obstacle: Lack of motivation

Solution: Motivation, like the body, must be fed often. Change your mindset and focus on things that build motivation, not destroy it. People, places, and things all affect motivation. Make a positive change if necessary.

Obstacle: Binge eating

Solution: Bingeing is often the result of starvation or lack of nutrients. Eating correctly throughout the day helps to ward off additional hunger. Bingeing also occurs when an emotional high or low (sedating feeling) is needed. Try consuming fruit in place of sweets. Initially, it's difficult, but once the fruit is eaten, the body is satisfied. In extreme cases, professional help is recommended.

Obstacle: Making wrong choices

Solution: We often make the wrong choice when we're very hungry; we'll eat anything that's within reach. Again, preplanned means prepared. Take healthy foods and store at work and at home. Think ahead what you'll eat, and plan accordingly.

One Step Ahead

Knowing what to expect in advance can dramatically affect your results. When you're aware, you're prepared. Stay a step ahead and prevent possible detours.

Take time and list three obstacles that could hinder your progress and how you'll prepare for them.

Example: You have an upcoming vacation or business trip, and you know you'll be eating out at least once a day.

Solution: Eat a light meal or healthy snack two to three hours before dining out. While dining out, commit to consuming only healthy foods in smaller portions. Very few restaurants have healthy food. Most use refined oils and the vast majority of options are not organic. If possible, check out the restaurant's online nutrition guide, and select what you'll order ahead of time. There are even websites that will help you choose the healthiest options at most chain restaurants.

Again, preparing for potential problems can prevent setbacks. When you do experience a step back, however, simply move forward. In the process, you're changing habits and, thus, a lifestyle. Research indicates that it takes approximately twenty-one days to establish a new habit. Set your sight on that target: new habits, new lifestyle.

Poor choices take us where we don't want to go, cost us more than we want to pay, and keep us longer than we want to stay.

CHAPTER FIVE

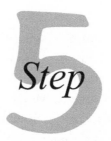

Step 5

Making the *Right* Choice

Food: friend and foe—
what you need to know

There are more books, articles, and journals currently written about food than at any other time in history, yet our problem with weight and poor nutrition continues to rise.

In the past, most health and diet consultants agreed on one point: caloric intake determines weight gain or loss.

Although new research points more to the type of food than daily caloric intake, I believe that both are important. Many people have not lost weight even when eating very healthy food. Often, it's because their daily caloric intake is too high. Beyond that, opinions vary concerning the types of calories to be consumed. Continually consuming more calories than you need will lead to weight gain— period! But on the flipside, counting calories is not the answer either.

What Does the Bible Say about Food?

The following section is an excerpt from my book, *Feasting and Fasting*:

There are many views regarding what diet is ideal. Vegans, vegetarians, proponents of plant-based diets, and meat promoters all argue that their diet is best. Throw the raw diet crowd into the mix, and the confusion only increases. Many of these diets overlap but with some stark differences. For example, hard-core raw advocates don't cook any food. They consume it straight from the tree, vine, or ground. Plant-based diets promote raw, but they are often flexible and have a much broader range of choices.

I don't claim to have all the answers. Even experts in the field of nutrition are divided, but again, we can glean a great deal from the biblical account. Most diets are written from an evolutionary perspective, so it's important that we get our facts straight. So let's begin where God begins.

In the beginning of creation, God said:

"Behold, I have given you every plant yielding seed that is on the surface of all the earth, and every tree which has fruit yielding seed; it shall be food for you; and to every beast of the earth and to every bird of the sky and to every thing that moves on the earth which has life, I have given every green plant for food"; and it was so. (Gen. 1:29–30 NASB)

We were designed to eat living, plant-based food. The life of the plant via vitamins, minerals, and enzymes is to be deposited into the body—to restore, renew, and replenish. We read that, after the flood, everything that lives and moves was to be food for us except the blood that is in the animal (Gen. 9:3). The blood of an animal contains toxins. Many diseases travel in the blood. God also identified clean and unclean animals. Unclean animals, such as pork, are still not considered healthy since viruses, bacteria, and parasites are easily transferred from the pig to us.

Was man not to consume meat until after the flood, approximately 1,600 years after the fall? If so, why? Did early man eat only plants for over sixteen centuries before God allowed meat?[21] How did a plant-based diet provide vitamin B12, calcium, iron, and zinc when they are difficult to obtain in a plant-based diet? Is it permissible to eat meat and dairy but not ideal? Should it be consumed sparingly? Does it balance nature (i.e., kill and eat)?

Biblically speaking, you can find support for a few different views, but we are encouraged to let our moderation be known to all men. Moderation means drinking or eating something occasionally. Unfortunately, moderation is often abused, and very unhealthy patterns develop. Paul said all things may be allowed, but all things are not beneficial (1 Cor. 10:23). In most areas where people live the longest, their diets are primarily plant-based.

I believe that the pre-flood atmosphere of the earth was much different than our living conditions today. Man lived in a healthier environment that may have provided more oxygen and greater protection against the harmful rays of the sun, and nutrient-dense plants and fruit-bearing trees grew in abundance. After the flood, however, fruits and vegetables became scarce (see Gen. 8:22: seedtime and harvest). I believe that God allowed meat consumption because of this scarcity. Healthy meat and dairy can be enjoyed from time to time for those who want to go this route, but it shouldn't be consumed in abundance. Personally, I'd rather err on the side of eating what we ate before the fall as my primary source of nutrition.

In short, I suggest consuming meat and dairy sparingly. Our main diet should consist of nutrient-dense foods such as legumes and potatoes (for those not limiting carbs), and big, colorful salads made with homemade dressing without sugar and refined oils.

Adaptation

It's also wise not to eat the same thing month in and month out. This avoids adaptation, which is when your body adapts or adjusts to what you're consuming. For example, adding healthy meat occasionally may help adjust hormone levels. Breaking up intermittent fasting days may also help because your body doesn't know what to expect. For example, if I eat a certain way for weeks and do the same exercises, my metabolism seems to slow down as my body adjusts and adapts to the consistent pattern.

God designed us in such a way that long-term caloric restriction will slow down our metabolism to help us survive. This is why most people hit plateaus. When the body thinks it's starving, it will adjust accordingly. The key isn't to eat *less* but to eat *less often*. Stop when you feel satisfied, not full. At the end of the day, you do, in fact, eat less calories, but this health hack prevents the body from thinking that you're starving. This is why being active is so important; you will burn even more fuel (calories). Fat is really just stored energy. Always look for opportunities to increase your activity.

These activities, in combination, can burn as much as 7,000 calories or more in a month and increase your metabolic rate. This could mean a two-pound loss or more within a month and a twenty-four-pound loss or more in one year. In addition to the caloric burn benefit, you'll develop healthier habits. Simply incorporating these few changes can also strengthen self-discipline in other areas and help to develop other character traits.

The NEAT Principle

One way to lose weight without much effort can be found in the *non-exercise activity thermogenesis* (NEAT) principle, which refers to the amount of energy (calories) burned for "everything we do that is not sleeping, eating, or sports-like exercise. It ranges from the energy expended walking to work, typing, performing yard work, undertaking agricultural tasks and fidgeting. Even trivial physical activities increase metabolic rate substantially."[22]

When you choose daily activities that are more active, you're increasing your NEAT and burning more calories overall. Watching television, playing video games, riding in a car, and surfing the web burn only 0–50 calories per hour, while climbing stairs, organizing closets, vacuuming, and washing your car burn over 100–200 calories per hour. In fact, "these high-effect NEAT movements could result in up to an extra 2000 [calories] of expenditure per day beyond the basal metabolic rate, depending on body weight and level of activity.[23] Therefore, daily making the choice to do one activity over another, such as walking to work rather than driving, increases your NEAT, and your body burns more calories.

I do realize there are those times when your body and mind need a rest, and television or movies can offer good entertainment. But keep it balanced. Taking one day a week to rest is recommended. I also encourage small breaks throughout the day.

Food Choices and Caloric Intake

When your body is short on energy (calories), it will draw from other sources for that energy. Your body will feed on stored tissue such as adipose (fat) tissue. Although I encourage seasons of fasting, starvation diets fail because they deplete the body of its needed energy source. Again, many diet books skip around the "calorie issue," saying that it's not necessary to worry about them. But I can truly say had I not kept an eye on my caloric intake, I would not have lost a significant amount of weight because I didn't realize how many calories I was consuming. However, it's easy to become obsessed with counting calories, which I do not recommend. Monitoring food intake should be used as an educational aid, not a lifelong obsession.

Many of America's most popular foods have little if any food value and a high calorie content. What's more, far too many people ignore the nutritional value of food. They are slowly undermining health because of poor food choices. The purpose of food is to meet our nutritional needs, not our wants!

As mentioned earlier, a controversial sweetener, aspartame, for example, is used in many products (e.g., diet drinks, yogurt, gum, meal replacement drinks, supplements). Research has shown that although aspartame is sweet, the adverse effects can be detrimental to health. Aspartame was discovered in 1965 when Dr. Schlatter, while working on an anti-ulcer medication, mixed a substance with methanol (wood alcohol). The result was a very sweet taste. The FDA has been reviewing this additive for many years, and the reports have been startling. Many animals, including roaches, won't consume it. Should we? You be the judge!

Today, more than ever, we're exposed to powerful food agents, additives, and enhancers. The list of controversial products we consume is sizeable. In all honesty, I'm surprised that we do not see more sickness and disease. Many people consume harmful foods for breakfast, lunch, and dinner—as well as snacks. For instance, how many times do people consume diet drinks or soft drinks instead of the water they need? The question isn't *if* these food choices can cause damage to the body but *when* they'll cause damage.

The Fear Factor

Through my experience in the fitness industry, I've found that many who begin a weight-loss program do so because of *fear*—fear of an early death, failing health, the onset of cancer, or other health-related illnesses. A high percentage of those I talk with who want to begin a weight-loss routine are already experiencing significant health problems. How sad that exercise and eating correctly are the last resort when they should be the first.

Many of our nation's diseases are related to nutrition. I can say without a doubt that, at present, poor nutrition is one of America's deadliest habits. It's a constant challenge because it's always before us. The American diet is socially acceptable, and the effects of poor nutrition, in many cases, are not recognized for some time. Unfortunately, we are unaware and unconcerned until our health is jeopardized. What a sad commentary on the lifestyle of a nation that has such great potential to live in the blessing God has so graciously given. I cannot stress enough the importance of ridding your lifestyle of these nonessential and often hazardous products, not only for you but for the next generation as well.

Quickly review the basics. Stick to organic, whole foods whenever possible. This is a simple list because, often, too much information can hinder progress. Remember, *less is more.* **The less complicated your lifestyle, the more control you'll have.**

Although meat is not essential to life, as vegetarians have shown, certain types of meat and especially clean fish, for example, are healthy and thus recommended in moderation occasionally. Many health experts also recommend raw organic dairy products.

The Real Deal on Carbohydrates

A calorie is a unit of energy derived from food. The energy comes from three main sources: *carbohydrates* (a source of energy for the body), *fats* (an essential nutrient for life-sustaining functions as well as an energy source), and *proteins* (used for building and repairing tissue and can be used as an energy source if other means are not available). All three are important in the weight-loss process.

Carbohydrates are currently at the forefront of most diet discussions. They consist of foods that originate from the ground (e.g., potatoes, whole grains, fruits, vegetables) and foods developed by man. Many people choose the wrong type of carbohydrates: those developed by man, such as sweets, processed foods, soft drinks, pastries, and white flour products.

Our bodies were designed to consume healthy, ground-originating carbohydrates, especially if you are very active. Many Scriptures found throughout the Bible refer to clean, God-given carbohydrates. Ezekiel 4:9, for example, states, "Also take for yourself wheat, barley, beans, lentils, millet, and spelt . . . and make bread for yourself." We are further encouraged to let our moderation be known to all men. The key word is *moderation*. Eat moderately, and keep in mind that even healthy foods should be consumed in moderation.

When we use energy through muscle exertion and cellular activity, we must replenish the energy, often with more carbohydrates. Therefore, certain carbohydrates aren't the enemy; overconsumption is.

After carbohydrates are consumed, they are broken down into glucose. One of three processes occur:

1. The glucose will serve an immediate need, such as exercise or activity, or assist in recovery.

2. If there is no immediate need, glucose (carbohydrate) is stored in the muscle and liver for future use.

3. If the liver and muscles are full, as they usually are in sedentary America, the glucose will be converted into fat and stored for future use. The storage capacity in the liver is rather small. It's used to supply energy to the brain and central nervous system, whereas, the storage capacity in the muscle is larger (more muscle means more storage capacity). Weight gain occurs when too many calories, mainly from the wrong type of carbohydrates, are consumed and not used.

The first and second processes are the most ideal. Again, carbohydrate consumption, in moderation and in the right form, is necessary. Consuming too many causes weight gain.

On average, individuals within our culture consume over 270 calories a day from refined sugar. Whether the source is a candy bar or a protein bar, it's still sugar. In refined form, these large doses, over time, are frequently responsible for failing health and obesity.

By decreasing nonessential sugar from 180 grams to 50 grams a day, caloric intake would decrease by 520 calories. One 12-ounce can of Coke, for instance, contains 35 grams of sugar and 140 calories. Theoretically, you could lose 1 pound a week by doing nothing more than deleting three-fourths of the refined, unhealthy sugar from your diet. Again, the type of sugar I'm referring to is the type found in soft drinks, coffee drinks, sweetened beverages, and sweets in general.

Many blame *all* carbohydrates for our nation's weight problem. As a result, low carbohydrate diets have become popular. While there are some good benefits, especially for those struggling with diabetes, we can't live in the ketogenic state forever, and extremely limiting healthy carbohydrates leaves little room for important fiber intake and healthy gut enzymes (think organic beans).

Most of these diets exclude whole grains and fruit and only allow vegetables. Doing this now and then has its benefits, but overall calorie consumption determines weight gain in most people, not carbohydrates. However, I agree that carbohydrates such as white bread, pastries, candy, soft drinks, and most fast foods should be minimized, if not eliminated. Health should always be the central factor when choosing a food or weight-loss program. Without health, a trim body has little significance!

Glycemic or Gimmick

The glycemic index (G.I.) has gained popularity in the weight-loss industry. The G.I. is an index chart that demonstrates the rate at which certain carbohydrates enter the bloodstream. A food low on the index has a slower rate of absorption. According to this theory, the slower the absorption rate, the lower the probability that it will be stored as fat in comparison to foods with high absorption rates. A carbohydrate high on the glycemic index can cause blood sugar levels to spike considerably. The higher the spike, the more insulin released into the bloodstream. This release of insulin tells the body to store fat.

Not everyone agrees with this theory because of confounding factors. For example, when eaten with other foods, the carbohydrate's rate of absorption can change significantly. Another problem with this index is that even though a food may have a slow rate of absorption, it is irrelevant if caloric intake is too high. Too many calories consumed will be stored as fat regardless of the rate of absorption. Granted, it is a good idea to eat foods with a slower absorption rate while also monitoring your caloric intake.

Fortunately, many natural foods have a slow absorption rate (e.g., nuts, some fruits, whole, unprocessed grains, most vegetables). If you're eating correctly, you won't need to pay close attention to this index unless you have a health-related illness that requires you to do so. Bodybuilders, diabetics, and fitness competitors, for example, do find this chart useful in helping to monitor and regulate blood sugar levels.

NOTE: The long-term consequence of high insulin levels is the possible development of diabetes. Diabetes is increasing every year and is among America's most pressing health concerns. Eating correctly is not only essential for weight loss but also for good health. Type 2 diabetes is a lifestyle disease that does not have to affect most people.

In summary, successful weight reduction depends on the foods you choose. Again, it's all about choices and making the right ones. Your body was designed to regulate the energy you consume and the energy you expend. It's a wonderful system that God designed, which is why it is so important to choose the foods He designed for it to run smoothly.

Dining Out

It's especially hard to monitor caloric intake when dining out. It is difficult to know how the food was prepared (e.g., with butter or oil). Additionally, many restaurants serve two or three times more food than what should be consumed. Eating out several times a week can hinder your progress unless you make wise choices. Before dining out, ask yourself, "Do I want to feel the brief pain of discipline during the meal or the nagging pain of regret after the meal?" This simple question can make it much easier to make the right choice.

The following tips for dining out can save over 1,000 calories per meal—yes, *per meal*:

1. Kindly instruct your waiter not to serve bread or chips beforehand (out of sight, out of mind). **Calories saved: 200 to 400**

2. Order salad dressing on the side, using only a minimal amount. Try dipping your fork (1 tablespoon equals approximately 120 calories, if the dressing is primarily oil). Avoid eating croutons. They contain unnecessary calories and have little food value. **Calories saved: 200 to 500**

3. Choose one main carbohydrate with your meal. For example, if you order a chicken sandwich, don't order pasta salad or beans; the bread is enough. But you can add low-fat soup, vegetables, or salad with light dressing. **Calories saved: 200 to 600**

4. Many restaurants add butter to meat when preparing it. This makes the meat juicier and richer in flavor (nothing tastes better than saturated fat). Ask the waiter to cook your meat without using butter or oil. **Calories saved: 200 to 300**

5. Order vegetables steamed and without butter. Do not order them sautéed. *Sautéed* is just another word for "saturated in fat." Low-

fat dressing, vinegar, or lemon may be used to enhance the flavor. **Calories saved: 200 to 400**

6. Eat a small meal two hours before you dine out. This will help to avoid overeating. **Calories saved: 500 to 1000**

7. When ordering, have the sauce, cheese, bacon, or mayonnaise removed. **Calories saved: 250 to 400**

If all else fails, and a meal contains a great deal of calories, eat half and take the rest with you. Eat until you are satisfied, not full.

But again, I'm not a fan of eating out very often. Many people associate dining out with overeating. It becomes an excuse to eat more. This type of thinking may have been acceptable fifty years ago when families rarely dined out, but now dining out has become commonplace. Many families eat out three, four, or even five times a week. This overindulgence can kill a weight-loss program—as well as health and wealth (it's expensive). Cut out dining out, and you'll be amazed at how much money you save.

Simplify for Success: Less Is More

As you formulate a plan, keep in mind that *fat free* simply means that the ingredients used contain no fat, yet many of these foods are still high in calories. Pay closer attention to the overall health benefits of the food rather than to carbohydrate or fat content.

Most people can eat carbohydrates such as yams, Ezekiel bread, brown rice, and so on as long as their total caloric consumption is strategic and they are active. The intentions of some low-carb diets may be good, and for some, these diets may bring success for a season, but for many others, they don't work long-term. Many diets focus on quick fixes, but they don't include long-term solutions to the overall problem. Most people want something easy to understand and easy to follow. The simpler the plan, the easier it is to carry out. Less is more! The less you have to think about, the more control you will have.

Eat God-given whole foods while limiting junk carbs, and incorporate intermittent fasting and block fasting (more than twenty-four hours) into your program.

Get Set to Offset Your *Set Point*

"It seems like my body is always working against me. Why is this?" In most cases, your body will try to return to its *maintenance level* (set point). I talked about this earlier in regard to adaptation. A maintenance level/set point is where your body ideally wants to keep itself, and it's usually not where you want it to be. Your weight, your percentage of body fat, and your lean body mass (LBM) are all affected and controlled by your maintenance level. Because of this, you are constantly at war with what your body wants and what you want.

Maintenance levels are often determined by genetic predisposition; however, lifestyle plays a key role in the overall success of a weight-loss program. Some spend an entire lifetime trying to put weight on, while others try to take it off. Both share the fact that their body is inclined to return to its set point.

When you eat less than what your body actually needs, it sends a message to your brain signaling for more food (hunger). If you control your appetite and do not overeat, your body will pull the energy that it needs from the adipose (fat) tissue and other sources. Again, if this is done consistently and over a significant period, you will lose weight. I'm not recommending that you starve yourself while fighting off hunger. I'm suggesting that you know the difference between wanting to eat and needing to eat and learn to eat highly satisfying, low-calorie, healthy foods. We live in a society where food is readily available. In many cases, we need to make a conscious effort not to overindulge.

Even without activity or exercise, your body will burn calories (energy) twenty-four hours a day, seven days a week; this is known as your resting metabolic rate, or RMR.

You glance at the fuel gauge in your vehicle to see if it needs fuel. The same is true for your body. It's wise to know when to fuel up (eat) and when to drive (burn the energy that was consumed). Don't get discouraged. It's not the fall that hurts—it's staying down that does. But, remember, if you fall, fall forward.

Plateaus

During a plateau, progress appears to stop, and no additional changes take place. While perhaps not evident externally, internally the benefits of exercise are still creating cardiopulmonary improvement. But to continue losing weight, you must break the plateau, and one of three things must occur: (1) fluctuate caloric intake and the type of food (e.g., limit carbs), (2) add intermittent fasting, or (3) increase the duration or intensity of the exercise or become more active throughout the day.

Increasing *duration* (time) signals the body to release more energy for fuel. Duration can be increased simply by adding an extra day of exercise to the routine or by adding ten to fifteen minutes to each daily workout. Initially, this should be enough to create change. If it does not occur within the first seven to ten days, increase the level of activity (e.g., quicker, faster). As a result of the increased duration, a caloric deficit is once again created.

Breaking through a Plateau

To better understand how the body works, let's discuss the effect that exercise and food consumption have on the body. In simpler terms, a temporary weight-loss standstill is called a plateau. Basically, it's time to make a change.

Stages of a Plateau

1. When food consumption is lowered, a caloric deficit is created, and it can slow your metabolism.

2. As you exercise, your heart and pulmonary system become more efficient.

3. As a result of the increased efficiency, your resting metabolic rate (RMR) lowers, and thus, fewer calories are burned.

4. As you continue to create a deficit and add exercise, your body

once again adapts to the changes. As a result, your body becomes more efficient, and you no longer burn as many calories as you once did. But that's ok—you are becoming physically fit as a result.

5. In addition to those above, the heavier a person is, the more calories they expend. For example, a 150-lb. man will burn fewer calories walking than a man weighing 300 lbs. who is walking the same distance and at the same speed. Therefore, as you lose weight, you may burn fewer calories than you once did.

This shouldn't be discouraging; rather, it should be very encouraging. This is a major accomplishment. Cardiopulmonary output is now functioning at a higher level, and health and weight loss can continue to be maximized.

Again, when a plateau occurs, more often than not, an adjustment will need to take place. Some people can remain in a plateau for months, possibly even years. They keep doing the same things expecting different results. Others may rarely encounter a plateau. However, if you're aware of the biological changes (previously explained) that are occurring within your body, you can make the needed adjustments.

Ironically, as I was writing this chapter, I noticed a caloric recommendation for dogs listed on a bag of dog food. This recommendation was made: "The following feeding guidelines are for adult dogs with moderate activity levels. These guidelines should be adjusted as needed to maintain optimal weight." Even veterinarians understand the importance of proper food intake. If it's important for a dog, how much more important is it for us and our children?

Protein, Carbohydrates, and Fat: Friends or Foes

PROTEIN

You may not only be burning glycogen (stored carbohydrates) and fat during a workout, unfortunately, you may also be burning muscle, especially if you're not receiving sufficient nutrients, calories, or protein. Muscle tissue is also a source of energy. Consuming sufficient amounts of protein as well as carbohydrates can aid in protecting your muscle from being broken down and converted to fuel.

If you doubt this, think about the physique of a long-distance runner as opposed to that of a sprinter. The long-distance runner is skinny and thin in appearance; the sprinter is muscular and larger. Why? The sprinter uses less muscular tissue as fuel than does the long-distance runner, mainly because the sprinter uses short bursts of energy to power his or her run. And glycogen, not muscle tissue or fat, is the main fuel source for explosive bursts of energy. Therefore, in my opinion, based on what I've observed, it's imperative to consume a sufficient amount of carbohydrates in addition to protein so the body has a primary fuel source and won't resort to muscle for fuel.

To clarify, exercise (both cardiopulmonary and resistance) increases the amount of protein needed for recovery, repair, and the building of new muscle. When calories are restricted or reduced, and sufficient carbohydrates and fats are not being consumed, protein (muscle) will be used for energy and not for its intended purpose of building and repairing.

More on Protein

When beginning, a good rule of thumb is to keep your daily protein intake around 20 percent of your total caloric intake for the day. Keto diet advocates will not be happy with this advice, but again, I'm writing from my experience based on working with many people over the years. And I'm writing to the average Joe, not the elite athlete. I actually do advocate higher protein recommendations in some cases, but 20 percent is a good rule of thumb to follow.

Note: 1 gram of protein equals 4 calories. A 4-ounce chicken breast, for example, contains approximately 187 calories and approximately 35.2 grams of protein. Therefore, 140 calories are derived from protein (35.2 x 4 = 140); the other 47 calories come from fat.

Below are my top personal choices for protein for meat eaters, and why:

1. Organic eggs

They are an excellent snack from time to time when hard-boiled ,and they combine easily with salads, tuna, and pasta. There are approximately 16 calories and 4 grams of protein per egg white. The yolk adds 50 calories, mainly from fat, but they are good to consume as well (choose organic, cage-free when possible).

I'm aware that cage-free doesn't always mean healthy, but we have to choose well when possible. When considering dairy, we must look at what the animals are consuming and, hopefully, that doesn't include GMO food. But it's often not possible to know what they're eating when they are roaming around the field. As stated earlier, this is why I recommend eating meat and dairy in moderation and eating very clean plant-based foods. I wish we could all farm our own land and milk our own cows, but that's not realistic for the majority of us.

3. Organic skinless chicken breast

Skinless chicken breast, still a favorite on most menus, has approximately 190 calories per 4-ounce serving and only 4 grams of fat. It also contains 35 grams of protein. When dining out, ask for a grilled 4-ounce chicken breast, cooked plain. Use hot sauce, salsa, low-fat sauces, or spices to add flavor.

4. Clean (not farmed) fish

Choices such as grilled tuna, salmon, or halibut are at the top of my list of favorites. They provide essential fats and are a great source of protein. Mediterranean diets (i.e., Greek, French, Italian) are rich in omega fatty acids and are some of the healthiest food choices. If you don't eat fish, add Omega-3 supplements to your program. Omega-3 is also found in flaxseed oil and walnuts. (Omega-6 is found in vegetable oils.)

For a Plant-based Diet

My top choices for protein on a plant-based diet (I aim for 85 percent plant-based foods in my diet) are plant-based protein powder and soaked beans (not canned when possible). Plant protein powder is easy to use. One scoop contains approximately 20 grams of protein and can be added to juice or milk. And organic beans on the side are a great source of fiber and protein and provide important gut enzymes. There is a misconception that meat protein is better than plant protein. It has to do with the amino acid complexities, but in a nutshell, when the animal eats plants, they get protein from the plants, which is assimilated into the muscle and consumed by us.

CARBOHYDRATES

Again, the types of carbohydrates that come from the ground and remain in their most natural state are essential to good health (e.g., whole grains, beans, vegetables, fruit). Our greatest problem is that we consume too many and the wrong types.

Listed below are my personal top four choices (organic, when possible) for carbohydrates and why:

1. One-half cup oatmeal (dry = 27 grams carbohydrates)

Oatmeal is a good source of fiber. Oatmeal satisfies longer than most breakfast choices.

2. One-half cup cooked pinto beans (22 grams carbohydrates)

Beans contain up to 8 grams of fiber per serving. They are rich in nutrients and tend to satisfy longer than other carbohydrates.

3. Bananas (27 grams carbohydrates)

I often add bananas to pancakes, french toast, low-fat cottage cheese, and other meals for flavor. Other fruit works just as well.

4. 1 cup sweet potatoes (27 grams carbohydrate)

No secret here—everyone loves potatoes. Alone, they tend to spike insulin levels. Adding healthy butter, broccoli, and lean meat to the meal, however, will offset the spike considerably.

Remember that a minimum of three to five servings of fruit and leafy vegetables daily is essential for optimum health. Most fruit and vegetables are low in fat and calories and high in nutrients. They're great for managing weight as well as health.

FAT

Fat (lipid) is a powerful source of energy. Rather than the kind of fat that you would find in a cheeseburger, I'm talking about the kind of fat found in nuts and avocados. Depleting this energy source hurts, not helps, the body.

Many nutritionists suggest that fat intake for the day should not exceed 20 to 25 percent of your daily caloric total unless you're trying the ketogenic approach for a season. In other words, if you're consuming 1,500 calories a day, no more than 300 to 360 of those calories, or 33 to 40 grams, should come from fat, according to some experts. My percentage is closer to 35 percent if I factor in avocados and nuts that I eat daily.

However, the amount of fat an individual should consume depends on whether they are carbohydrate sensitive (hypoglycemic). Many who are may find it helpful to increase their fat intake to 40 percent (while keeping saturated at the lower end) for optimal performance. Others may lower it to 15 percent, depending on how their body reacts. For example, I feel incredible after a large salad with a small chicken breast and avocado compared to the same amount of calories from a healthy homemade cheese pizza with organic ingredients. I can tell the difference, therefore, I eat accordingly.

Special note: I often make my own salad dressing from the juice of organic pepperoncinis. Good recipes can be found online. Making your own salad dressings allows you to avoid refined oils. When I use the word *refined*, it means that nutrients are removed and chemicals are added, especially in the case of oils. Refined vegetable oils are often sold in bulk and end up in many prepackaged food items—even healthy ones.

Once heated to high temperatures, they are then processed with petroleum solvents and heated again to remove waxy buildup. More chemicals are then added to remove the smell. Long term, they can wreak havoc on our body and fuel both disease and inflammation. Many attribute heart disease to refined vegetable oils for this very reason. Whether it's sugar, refined oil, or processed food, junk is the main culprit in our nation's massive health crisis.

Are You Carbohydrate Sensitive?

Those who suffer from hypoglycemia are often carbohydrate sensitive because they're eating too much sugar. If they eat the wrong combinations of food (depending on the severity of the condition) adverse reactions can occur. If you're not sure if you're carbohydrate sensitive, here are a few clues:

- you crave sweets after eating meals containing carbohydrates

- you feel irritable or lethargic if you don't eat frequently

- you feel sleepy after a few hours of not eating

- simple sugars (e.g., some fruit, table sugar) make you jittery

- during certain times of the day you feel dizzy, or as though you could pass out

Your doctor can request a glucose tolerance test to determine if you are hypoglycemic and offer suggestions to help. Here are a few ideas that helped me:

- Develop a healthy eating pattern.

While weaning off of processed sugar, I occasionally use a little Manuka honey or maple syrup. Granted, I don't follow a perfect regime every day, but I do get back on track as often possible. For example, as I was writing this chapter, my daughter came home from church and handed me a cookie. Instead of turning it down, I had a bite with her, and we had a great time.

You have to set boundaries more often than not, but please also be flexible. There are exceptions, though. For example, if you have a health crisis, it may be time to buckle down and make some hard decisions and say no to food as long as it takes. A year ago, our church fed the homeless, and we provided meals. I ate fried chicken and pizza with them, then got back on track the next day. It's not about legalism. It's about using wisdom and making more right choices than wrong choices. (On that note, I really wish we would feed the less fortunate better food in our nation and not give them cheap products.)

- Include fiber at every meal.

- Choose carbohydrates such as whole grains and oat bran but primarily vegetables.

- Try not to consume carbohydrate-only meals.

- Incorporate regular workout times into your lifestyle.

- Plan for seven hours of sleep each night. Shut off the media in the evenings, and let your body shut down and wake up on its own whenever possible.

- Use high-potency multivitamins and minerals regularly.

- Consume 1/2 to 1 gallon of water each day. Fill the container first thing in the morning and try to consume it by the end of the day. Again, clean water is the best choice.

Fat in moderation is desirable for healthy living. It helps to slow the digestion process and thus lessen the amount of insulin that is released into the bloodstream. Fat also creates a feeling of fullness. However, a popular bacon cheeseburger contains a whopping 1,000 calories and 55 grams of fat—this is not a good choice!

Listed below are my personal top four choices for fat, and why:

1. Raw almonds, 1 to 1-1/2 ounces (15 grams fat).

Almonds can be added to your favorite salad, morning cereal, and more. Be careful not to overindulge. Consume 1/2 an ounce (approximately 10 almonds) two or three times a day.

Keep in mind that most almonds in California are pasteurized and those that contain salt usually contain unhealthy salt and also added oil so that the salt sticks to the almonds.

2. Olive or coconut oil, 1 teaspoon (4 grams fat)

Olive oil is healthy and contains 2 grams of saturated fat per tablespoon.

3. Avocados, 1 ounce (5 grams fat)

This is another healthy fat. Add to salads and sandwiches.

4. Organic ghee: clarified butter, where solid fats have been skimmed off.

Plan Ahead

Planning ahead can save time and money as well as calories.

➤ Develop a master shopping list that you can reference online.

➤ Don't shop when hungry.

➤ Arrange a weekly menu plan.

➤ Repeat favorite menus often. Many times, we make the wrong choices because we don't have time to prepare a meal. By planning in advance, you can prevent the "grab it and eat it" syndrome.

➤ Plan the night before for the following day, or at least think it through. You'll be prepared. It's truly that simple.

➤ Plan on missing a meal or two a day and avoid snacking.

➤ One of the greatest helps, in many cases, is to plan on cutting your portions in half.

➤ A big help for our family has been to have pre-made salads available in large mason jars. Pour them in a bowl and add healthy dressing, and you're good to go.

Metabolism: Does It Really Matter?

We're often guilty of eating too much food at one time, *our metabolism thus smolders rather than burns.* Our bodies require small portions of food throughout the day to run efficiently. Additionally, your body can adapt to your new lifestyle changes, causing you to hit a plateau. It's called adaptation. If you hit a stall in your program, don't give up; understand that the body has adapted to what you're doing

,and you'll have to increase the intensity of your exercise, exercise more, or change your diet around and include intermittent fasting (more in chapter 6).

The size of our stomach is rather small. It was designed to hold a certain amount of food. Once that food is broken down and utilized, our brain sends a message to eat again, which is normally within two to four hours after the prior meal, provided that our previous meal was consumed in moderation.

Some say that eating small, frequent meals gives the body exactly what it's asking for—no more, no less— and that it keeps our metabolism running at a faster rate. That was the thought two decades ago, but new research shows that intermittent fasting and not eating throughout the day is now the best approach, and I believe that it's biblical.

I Barely Eat—Why Can't I Lose Weight

What about those individuals who don't eat much during the course of a day? Why do they have a hard time losing weight? First, it's important to know exactly how many calories are being consumed. Again, most people underestimate their caloric intake by over 40 percent. That's almost half the next day's calorie requirement. Don't get discouraged, that doesn't mean you need to eat less—just eat smart.

Five reasons why people fail in dieting.

1. They overlook dead calories in juice, coffee drinks, or soft drinks.

2. They snack throughout the day (*a little here, a little there* adds up).

3. They failure to realize how many calories are in certain foods and why dead foods are counterproductive.

4. They eat too many "healthy foods." (*Healthy* does not necessarily mean good for you).

5. They fail to move often (exercise and activities should be lifelong).

I often found that those who consumed only a small amount of calories Monday through Thursday used pills, coffee, diet soft drinks, or willpower to avoid overeating. However, they would binge over the weekend, snacking and consuming large meals that consisted of double portions of meat, carbohydrates, dessert, and alcohol. Just one of these weekend meals could consist of well over 1,500 calories or more. (I estimate that on Thanksgiving many people eat between 6000 and 8000 calories.)

Even though the caloric intake was low Monday through Thursday, nearly double the number of calories was consumed on the other three days. The metabolic rate, in response to what the body sensed as starvation, slowed down considerably and adapts. Most calories consumed were stored as fat because the body sensed that a period of starvation was pending. (I followed this pattern myself for many years until I realized that I did not see any significant progress, not to mention the damage it may have done to my body.)

Many people eat approximately 40 percent more calories each week than what they had assumed they'd eaten. They quickly find that dieting a few days a week is not the answer, so they give up and blame the diet. Again, diets don't work. Eating the right food and staying active does work. If nutrition is lacking, your metabolism cannot do its job effectively.

Note: Some people who don't binge on the weekends instead binge in the evenings. They may fail to eat breakfast and lunch but make up for it in the evening. When this occurs, the same principle applies—the body senses starvation and slows down.

Don't Allow a *Step Back* to Become a *Setback*

Throughout this chapter, one common theme was discussed: It's impossible to lose weight if more calories are consumed than are burned. This doesn't mean that you should consume 6,000 calories a day and follow it with a 10-hour jog. Nor does it mean that you should starve yourself. The key is to find out what works for you and stick with it. Again, I'm not advocating a calorie-counting diet—I'm advocating long-term awareness of the type, amount, and value of the food you're consuming. The key is not necessarily to eat less but to eat less often. Not all calories are equal. Our metabolic rate (the rate at which our body converts energy), hormone levels, lifestyle choices, and many other factors come into play. A person can eat 2,500 calories of junk food all day and gain weight, while another can consume 2,500 of God-given healthy food and maintain their weight. Dr. Daniel Pompa wrote a great article about this topic entitled "The Truth About Diet Restriction and Weight Loss."[24]

Caloric intake of the right foods is one of the most significant success factors, but it's also the most challenging part of any weight-loss program. Of the thousands of people I've helped to lose weight, none ate perfectly or exercised every day. However, they learned to make more right decisions than wrong ones and eventually developed a healthier, more energetic lifestyle. It's truly that simple.

I often encourage people to eat correctly at least 80 percent of the time. The problem is that after most people blow it a day or two in a row, they give up, and the "decision" to quit defeats success. Don't allow the word *quitting* to enter your mind. Remember, this is a lifestyle for the rest of your life.

Another essential part of health and weight management is learning how to manipulate indicators that cause you to eat. For example, after-dinner snacks always signaled me to overeat (for others, it may be social events, TV in the evening, or weekend get-togethers). As I became aware of this problem, my focus shifted from wanting to eat to needing to eat. I also ate more healthy, God-given food, which curbed my appetite for sweets.

Are You Off Course?

Analogies often help to clarify a principle. Let's view weight loss as a journey. You've left your home and have driven ten miles. You shift your car into reverse and drive backward one mile. It's not the direction you're going, but it doesn't take you all the way back home.

Again, many people, after slipping a day or two in a row, or even a week or two, act as if all their hard work was meaningless, and they quit. They allow a temporary problem to control a long-term decision.

During a successful weight-loss journey, everyone travels in reverse occasionally, but they don't drive back home. Successful people understand that one lost mile is not all ten! Even if you've been in reverse for ten miles, get back on track, and continue forward! Don't let a step back become a setback! And make sure to read my other two health-related books that can help in this area: *Feasting and Fasting* and *HELP! I'm Addicted.*

Are You Fit?

As mentioned earlier, those who are in great shape rarely, if ever, mention dieting. Fitness for them had become a lifestyle. Fitness describes the healthy interwoven condition of the body, mind, and spirit. It comes from the word *fit*, meaning to be in good health. We often judge a person's level of fitness by the way they appear on the outside. It's possible to appear fit on the outside and be far from fit on the inside. Fitness is not about following a diet and a special exercise program but about a lifestyle of someone who has a healthy relationship with God.

You can make that change today. It begins with a decision—a decision to change your lifestyle, to further your education, to spend more time with your family, and to do what it takes to lose the weight. Everything begins and ends with a decision. Decide today, and change tomorrow—and don't allow step backs to become setbacks.

When We Make a Decision, It Then Makes Us!

By following these simple guidelines, you will be moving closer to your goal and building a healthier lifestyle. Remember, it's easier to stick with a routine than it is to wing it every day. When you develop a routine, the routine becomes a habit, and habits develop into a lifestyle. As a result, new habits are developed, and weight loss is more easily achieved and maintained.

Work to incorporate healthy habits and remove the harmful ones.

Although there are weekly challenges, many find that better choices are easier to make because their desire to maintain a sense of well-being fuels their motivation. Desire will find a way, but excuses will hide the way. For example, in the past, I made excuses to avoid eating fruit and vegetables, so I'd ignore them altogether. Now I often take fruit, broccoli, cauliflower, carrots, and low-calorie dip to work in a lunch bag. That way, I have no other alternative but to eat them. Not only does this assure that my daily intake of fresh vegetables is met, but it gives me a mental boost to know I'm doing something good for my body.

Enduring truth: We make a decision; it then makes us

It's true that we make a decision and it then makes us. The choices we make will determine our level of success. The single decision to lose weight is easy, but daily making the right choices can, at times, be difficult. And it can be equally challenging to make correct choices without proper information. Thus, it is essential to seek accurate advice about your weight-loss process.

Wisdom directs that we seek counsel, but where we find that counsel from is vitally important. If we acquire information from misleading infomercials and slick marketing campaigns, we may be ill-advised. Granted, a few infomercials, advertisements, and other forms of soliciting are beneficial and do provide a certain degree of information, but to rely solely on that information is not wise. Seek advice from those who genuinely want to help and have accurate information.

Thoughts become words, words become actions, actions become habits, and habits determine our lifestyle.

CHAPTER SIX

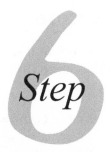

Step

Prioritizing Your Life

Overcoming the struggle within

W e've discussed choosing to change, wisdom, discipline, preparation, and choices. Prioritizing is the next important step. Prioritizing is the ability to apply properly first things first to your weight-loss program.

For those of you who exercise, generally, only 1/24th of your day will be spent exercising. That's a very insignificant amount of time, considering that many use seven hours a day just to sleep. As stated before, success is a result of an overall lifestyle, not how much time you spend exercising. Many individuals exercise regularly, up to five or six times a week, but their appearance does not change. Their overall lifestyle is the issue. When proper diet meets proper rest and a healthy relationship with God, it equals success. Granted, there are individuals who, through no fault of their own, cannot make diet changes. I'm assuming that the reader understands that I'm talking to those who can.

The Number One Excuse

You might be surprised at some of the excuses I've heard, but I'm sure you won't be surprised to learn that time is the number one excuse—and sometimes it's a good one.

Time is one of the most valuable commodities that you possess. It can thrust you into the core of achievement, or it can leave you consumed with guilt and regret. Time, if left to itself, will be the thief that robs you of opportunity, but when controlled, it can be used to great advantage. Use time wisely; it cannot be replaced!

I want to challenge those people who, like myself, do have the time to eat correctly and exercise. We often forget just how precious time is. How many days, weeks, or even months do we waste because we don't prioritize our lives? We need to be very careful when we say that we don't have enough time. What we are really saying is that it's not important. If it were, we would find the time. If we don't schedule time, time will schedule us.

You'll never get everything done that needs to be completed in a day. Therefore, you must prioritize your day. Ask yourself, "What's the most important thing for me to do in any given hour?" It's all about leading a productive, balanced life, and using time wisely. Don't let time be the excuse that stops you from succeeding. Your desire will find a way to lose weight, but excuses will hide the way.

Contrary to what many think, exercise can help with the utilization of time. With exercise, energy, enthusiasm and self-esteem often improve. When these areas run at peak performance, success dramatically increases! Social life, business life, spiritual life, and personal life all benefit from increased productivity! For example, employees who exercise are less likely to call in sick and are more productive while at work.

One of the more startling facts revealed in recent studies is that the average American family watches over seven hours of media a day. Yes, *seven hours*. That statistic alone is reason enough to reconsider how we spend our time. Time is not like money; it can't be borrowed, saved, or earned. You can, however, spend it—so spend wisely.

Which Is Best: Cardiopulmonary or Resistance Training?

Should I walk on the treadmill, climb a Stairmaster, or lift weights? This was perhaps one of the most frequently asked questions when I worked in fitness facilities. First, consider that we are less active today than at any other time in history. We move less, but we consume more. These key factors, less and more, when applied in reverse order—less "bad" food consumption and more activity—would aid in preventing obesity and related illnesses. There is a definite need to prioritize and include exercise in our daily routine.

With our modern age of technology came a lack of mobility. Most everything is designed with comfort and convenience in mind. A day's work often means sitting at a desk glued to a computer and burning a measly 60 to 80 calories per hour. Many years ago, we moved more at work and throughout the day. As a result, we burned more calories. The only logical answer is to increase our mobility through exercise—but which ones?

Resistance Training for Results

I want to encourage those of you who will not exercise with weights to at least incorporate some type of exercise into your weight-loss program (e.g., swimming, walking, biking). Many believe that riding a bike or walking on a treadmill is better than weight training for fat loss, but that's not necessarily true. Weight training, also known as *resistance training*, also aids in body fat reduction.

Trainers promote weight lifting because it builds lean body mass. Lean body mass (LBM) is comprised of muscle, bone, fluid, and other tissue. Lean body mass burns more calories than does adipose (fat) tissue. For example, a person with 150 pounds of lean body mass can burn more calories per day than a person with only 100 pounds of LBM. Muscle is one of the best calorie-burning tools available. Therefore, build muscle to burn more calories.

Muscle is broken down when we work out, then it builds up when we sleep and rest. We must feed it the right fuel, as well as get enough rest and find ways to relieve stress. And women, don't worry about looking like a big bodybuilder. Most of them take performance-enhancing drugs. Trust in the way that God designed you. You will not build enormous muscles. When you build muscle, the body also breaks it down and keeps you in a healthy state. Those on performance-enhancing drugs use those drugs to prevent muscle breakdown or add to muscle growth.

Those who are concerned about blood sugar levels, such as diabetics, should consider this. As we learned earlier, the majority of carbohydrates are stored in the muscle. Therefore, the more muscle one has, the more carbs can be stored. As we age, we lose muscle. Consequently, the body loses a percentage of its carbohydrate storage tanks. As a result, blood sugar levels may increase because the glucose that was once stored in the muscle is now recirculating through the liver, causing a rise in blood sugar. Incorporating resistance training into your weekly schedule can help to lessen this occurrence.

You can still lose weight and stay fit even if you choose not to lift weights, but together, weight training and cardiopulmonary training provide the ideal form of exercise. The adage is true: "If you don't use it, you will lose it." Many have overlooked resistance training simply because they were unaware of its significant role in body-fat reduction. For example:

- A twenty-minute leg workout can burn up to 300 calories.

- A forty-minute upper body training session can burn 300, 400, or more calories depending on the intensity, not to mention the post-exercise metabolic increase that also burns calories.

Sets and Repetitions

A set is a *group* of repetitions. For example, a leg curl performed in eight sequential movements could be considered one set and referred to as *1 set of 8 repetitions (reps)*. In my opinion, there's often too much attention given to exact sets and reps. Just take your body to a point where you can feel it.

Many people perform large numbers of reps and sets without properly exhausting the muscle. They focus on quantity rather than on quality. Some find that their best workouts consist of only two or three sets and up to 20 or 30 repetitions per set. Others find that two or three sets of 10 to 12 repetitions work better. Either way, I recommend performing the movement slowly, while keeping the muscle in a constant state of tension. By slowly controlling the movement, other muscles, as well as the primary muscle, are properly exhausted. When muscles are working properly to balance and support the movement, you are burning more calories because both the muscular and neurological systems are adapting to the unfamiliar workload, especially for beginners. That's why those who first begin a weight-lifting routine see noticeable strength gains within the first few weeks. The neurological system, in addition to the muscular system, is becoming accustomed to the new demand placed on it. As the neurological system adapts, strength immediately increases.

Repetition refers to "time under tension" (how much time the muscle is under the tension of the exercise being performed). For example, an arm curl taking only 3 seconds to perform and an arm curl taking 10 seconds to perform (i.e., 4 seconds up, hold for 2 seconds, 4 seconds down) are both considered a repetition. But the 10-second arm curl has a much longer period of "time under tension"; therefore, the muscle is being worked much harder.

In short, muscles are stimulated by movements and workloads they're not familiar with. Theoretically, the more unfamiliar the movement, the more adaptation will take place. Adaptation is what causes muscle growth, strength, and/or maintenance. The muscle, in response to the workload, will develop and strengthen to facilitate future demand. Mixing up your workout program is essential to long-term success, as is rest. Although muscle is broken down when we exercise, it develops when we rest.

So how many reps and sets should I do?

Again, it all depends on the workload and intensity, but a good rule of thumb is...

- For larger muscle groups (back, chest, legs), three to four exercises per body part consisting of two sets of 10 to 12 repetitions per set are sufficient.

- For smaller muscle groups (arms, shoulders), two to three exercises per body part consisting of two sets of 15 repetitions per set are sufficient.

If I've lost you with this example, don't worry—as long as you're stimulating the muscle, reps and sets aren't as important as many think. But you'll want to begin by doing very few of each, possibly only one set of 10.

Understanding Cardiopulmonary Training

Cardiorespiratory training, also known as *cardiopulmonary* training, is sometimes considered a form of resistance training. Cardiopulmonary training may be the most misunderstood form of exercise because many believe that only fat is being burned, when in reality that may not be the case.

Cardiopulmonary training assists fat loss by helping to create a caloric deficit. Additionally, there are many associated health benefits. When you ride a bike, for example, your body will require a certain amount of energy to carry out the activity. If the bike ride requires 600 calories of energy to fuel the activity, many experts suggest that your body will first take from your glycogen (carbohydrate) storage for the fuel it needs. After ten to fifteen minutes of continued biking, your body will resort to a more evenly distributed energy-burning process. It will then burn both glycogen and adipose tissue (fat) for the fuel that it needs (muscle may also be used as fuel if proper nutritional guidelines aren't followed or if the exercise is intense or exceeds an hour in length).

A caloric deficit will then be created as long as your caloric consumption does not exceed your caloric expenditure (outflow). When output exceeds input, change will occur. However, as we discovered earlier, if sufficient amounts of calories are not being consumed, some muscle may be converted and used for energy. That's why many who lose weight also lose muscle. As a result, strength decreases considerably, and although weight loss has occurred, the overall tone of the body has remained soft. The reason is that both fat and muscle, along with glycogen, were used as energy during the weight-loss program.

Are You Burning Muscle?

There have been many questions raised about the body's ability to burn muscle during cardiopulmonary exercise. Starvation diets can force the body to use muscle for fuel, but intermittent fasting, and even long-term fasting, can put the body into what is called a "protein-sparing" phase, where large amounts of muscle are spared because fat becomes the primary source of fuel (ketosis). God knew what He was doing by sparing the muscle and utilizing fat during fasting. If your body is not getting enough fuel (food), it will not shut down like a vehicle, but it will find another fuel source—some muscle but primarily fat.

We generally want to experience quick results, and we tend to think "more is better." However, working out is stressful on the immune system, especially if the body is not allowed enough time to rest. The harder you push, the more rest you'll need. Granted, this is hard to regulate. Listen to your body, rest when you need rest, and exercise when you need exercise.

For example, an hour cycling class can burn a tremendous number of calories (600 to 1,000). A 30-minute jog on a treadmill can burn between 300 and 400 calories. Your body would require more rest and nutrition after intense cycling as opposed to an easy jog on the treadmill. Again, intensity plays a key role in the number of calories burned as well as the recovery time needed after the exercise.

Eight Choices to Help Avoid Overtraining

➤ Exercise when energy levels are at their peak for the day.

➤ Eat a small meal one or two hours before your workout if you must, but intermittent fasting works well for me. For example, I will begin my workout routine after 14 hours of fasting with a tremendous amount of energy, but this must be built up to. The old thought, "Don't work out in the morning on an empty stomach unless you are conditioned to do so." may be true for many people who have not yet conditioned themselves.

➢ Be very sensitive to overexertion. If you're exhausted, consider taking a break.

➢ If possible, eat a balanced meal within an hour after you work out to replenish and restore the energy that was lost and the nutrients that might be deficient, such as amino acids.

➢ Work out with weights first, a minimum of 20 minutes and a maximum of 45. Next, perform cardiopulmonary exercises, a minimum of 20 and a maximum of 40 (this routine is for weight loss.) However, I sometimes do cardiovascular training first, or I mix it around. Some of my best workouts have focused on 10 to 15 minutes of high-intensity cardiovascular training followed by 15 minutes of weight training, back to cardiovascular training.

➢ If you can't work out with weights first, alternate your weight-training days and your cardiopulmonary-training days (e.g., weights on Monday, treadmill on Tuesday, weights on Wednesday)

➢ Work out a minimum of 3 days a week and a maximum of 6 for those already conditioned.

➢ When beginning, work your upper body one day and your lower body the next, with one day off in between.

Exercise is not the same as "working all day." People often believe that they don't need exercise because they perform physical work all day. Unless your job includes walking three miles a day at a fast pace, nonstop or working a physical job, you probably need to exercise. Again, the intensity of the exercise is a huge factor in determining caloric expenditure.

High-intensity workouts (e.g., jogging for five minutes, sprinting for one, repeating for twenty minutes) produce a greater amount of *excess post-oxygen consumption* or EPOC, which is the *after-burn effect* of exercise. More intense workouts produce more post-oxygen consumption. In other words, if Meredith jogs and sprints for twenty minutes, while Diane walks for twenty minutes, not only is Meredith burning more calories during the exercise but she's also going to burn more after exercising due to the higher utilization of oxygen.

Breaking the Exercise Plateau

In addition to caloric-intake plateaus discussed earlier, you may also hit a plateau as the result of exercise. Exercise causes the body to make many changes within the cellular structure. These changes use energy, or more calorie expenditure. Once the body adjusts to the changes, the energy that was once needed is no longer needed. As a result, metabolism slows to accommodate the effects that exercise is having on the body, and less caloric expenditure occurs.

The more we exercise, the more our bodies become conditioned or accustomed to it. As a result, we use fewer calories than we once did. Many become frustrated and stop exercising because they no longer see results. If this happens, adjust your workout. As we discussed earlier, begin by either increasing your workout intensity or your workout duration.

If you've been exercising for three consecutive months or more, it's best to stop exercising for a week to allow your body to break through the adaptation phase, but don't quit exercising altogether. Exercise is not only good for weight loss but for overall health as well.

What about Target Heart Rate?

The Target Heart Rate (THR) chart measures the rate at which the cardiopulmonary system is working. You'll want to exercise hard enough to expend sufficient amounts of energy without exerting yourself beyond an acceptable range. There are ways to determine your THR, but I've found the simplest, most effective way for beginners is the Talk Test:

- If you can carry on a conversation while exercising, your level of exertion is too low. Either increase the *speed* or the *level* at which the exercise is being performed.

- If you can't say a few words without gasping for air, lower the intensity to a reasonable level. You should be able to speak a short sentence without panting for breath.

The Yo-Yo Effect

The majority of people who lose weight on a "diet" gain it back within two years while adding more weight. Don't get discouraged by this. They generally had short-term diet goals and, thus, no long-term results. You think you'll be different, right? Briefly stated, here's how the yo-yo effect works:

During an unrealistic, restrictive diet, many fail to consume enough protein and calories to sustain the required levels of lean body mass (LBM). The lack of calories for fuel causes the body to burn muscle in conjunction with fat and carbohydrates for energy, especially if sufficient amounts of protein are not being consumed. (We do not want this.) Muscle is a calorie-burning machine. If we starve it away, we will severely hinder the weight-loss process.

As the body recognizes that calories are being restricted, it forces the metabolism to slow down and thus burn fewer calories. When caloric intake is severely limited, not only does your body burn muscle but it adjusts to the changes by not burning as many calories as it once did. As a result, your brain signals for food, and hunger is dramatically increased. Weight is regained, and more is added to prepare for any future starvation.

Note: Consuming 10 to 20 percent below your maintenance level to lose weight is not starving the body, severely restricting calories and nutrients is. Additionally, those who incorporate intermittent fasting into their lifestyle rarely gain back a lot of weight.

Preventing the Yo-Yo Effect

1. Incorporate lasting lifestyle changes — don't diet!

2. Avoid starvation and unrealistic diets; the fastest way is not the best way. But keep in mind that intermittent fasting and seasons of long-term fasting are not starvation. You're simply switching

the energy source and cleaning your body from the inside out (more in chapter 8).

3. Consume ample amounts of plant-based foods, such as colorful vegetables, per meal. It not only adds a tremendous amount of nutrient-dense food to your diet but it also curbs your appetite for unhealthy things.

4. Try to fast one day a week.

5. Don't make poor short-term decisions that have long-term consequences.

6. Don't use caffeine or stimulants to control appetite. Allow the body to operate the way it was designed.

7. Eat to live rather than live to eat. Remember that health is your primary focus.

More on Low-Carbohydrate Diets

In the last two decades, we have seen the benefit of minimizing carbs, but many low-carbohydrate diets severely restrict the consumption of whole grains, beans, and fruit. Initially, low-carbohydrate diets will result in a more significant loss in weight (4 to 8 pounds), but not *fat weight*. The weight that is initially lost when cutting back on carbohydrates is comprised of fluid, protein (muscle), and fat. Increased hunger can be associated with low-carbohydrate diets.

I cannot give a one-size-fits-all approach because some people need to use a ketogenic method for a season, while others need to focus on healthy, life-giving carbohydrates. What are your goals, and what are you trying to accomplish? How much weight do you need to lose, and what type of medical conditions do you have? These types of questions and many more must be taken into consideration before making severe diet changes. For most people, they simply need to rid their diet of bad carbohydrates such as crackers and chips and countless other things and add nutrient-dense carbohydrates such as beans and large salads. I don't see any harm in a person having a cup of organic beans with their salad.

More Important than Food and Exercise

Although exercise and correct food intake are essential, they alone do not guarantee results. What you feed your mind is just as critical and probably more important than what you feed your body. Our most difficult battles are within. Every action we take, or fail to take, begins with a thought. Thoughts will talk us out of and into every decision that we'll make. How many times have you stopped yourself from succeeding because of the limitations created by a thought? Most Americans are aware that health and fitness should be a top priority, but they still do little or nothing about it. Their ideas, especially of long-term commitment, discourage them.

Nations were born and companies established because someone's thought became action. Your mind is the most powerful tool that you possess. It can stop you from overeating, or it will allow the excess. It will awaken you at five in the morning to work out, or it will tell you to sleep in. It will keep you focused, or it will distract you. Many people fail before they even begin because their thoughts limit them. Your thoughts become words, your words become actions, your actions become habits, and your habits become your lifestyle!

That's a powerful principle. It's your choice, your decision, your outcome. What you focus on, you will get. Do your actions and habits produce the positive results you want? If not, change the way you think. As a result, your actions and habits will follow.

Who you are on the inside will determine who you are on the outside. Many people do not finish what they start because internal, as well as external, obstacles discourage them. Being aware that there will be setbacks mentally and physically and being equally prepared to move forward regardless will eventually take you where you want to go.

Life does not have to control you. *You* cannot change what happens to you, but you can control how you respond to it. Again, a step back is not a setback unless you refuse to move forward!

Realistic Expectations

Are your expectations realistic? Unrealistic expectations, according to psychologists, are major contributors in relational as well as many other problems. Unrealistic expectations can also hinder your weight-loss program. If expectations are not realistic, weight loss will become increasingly more difficult.

Earning a degree can take years of dedication, education, determination, and perseverance. One doesn't merely show up, pick up their doctorate, and leave. They complete the work necessary to receive the degree. The same is true for weight loss. We can't eat whatever we want, whenever we want, take a pill, and expect good results. Like it or not, there is no shortcut to lifelong success in weight management—you must remain consistent. Once you change patterns, your lifestyle will be self-generating and your greatest asset in helping you maintain enthusiasm and continued success. Again, energy creates energy.

There is no formula that states how much weight you will lose or by when. Everyone loses weight differently. One thing is certain: The more structured and disciplined you are, the faster the results.

Note: As your body adapts to these changes, the amount of weight you lose will rise and fall depending on genetic predisposition, lifestyle, metabolism, and the biological changes that are taking place within the body.

Enduring truth: Prioritizing—putting first things first

Prioritizing means "putting first things first." Getting and staying fit is crucial, but sometimes tricky. This shouldn't surprise us. Proverbs 14:23 says, "In all labor there is profit, but idle chatter leads only to poverty." *Labor* is another word for *effort; idle* is another word for *inactivity.* In simpler terms, effort produces results; inactivity doesn't! Putting first things first leads to success. Those things in life worth having, including weight loss, generally take energy and commitment to achieve.

Don't be discouraged if you're not where you want to be. Again, the secret is learning to make more right choices than wrong ones and to rise each time you fall. Begin again, and move forward. Perseverance is your greatest attribute at this time.

Those who succeed walk through adversity, not without it!

CHAPTER SEVEN

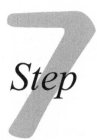

Step

Lifestyle Changes that Last

Maintaining your results
(It's not as hard as you may think)

Perhaps you feel like you've failed in the past when trying to change your lifestyle. Don't forget one major theme of this book: Forget what lies behind, and press ahead. Begin now initially, or begin again. Success doesn't come without failure. It's through our failures that we learn how to succeed. They often make us more determined. Remember, successful people fail more than unsuccessful people do; they just begin again.

Don't think that weight loss is difficult to achieve. That's not the case. Focused attention, knowledge, planning, working your plan, and rising each time you fall determines victory. Again, we make it more difficult than it is by not adhering to basic age-old principles of success: persistence, patience, discipline, and consistency. The secret to success has not changed; we've changed. But don't let these four words scare you. You are persistent, patient, disciplined, and consistent in some areas of your life—simply apply them to others.

One of the most disheartening statistics about weight loss is that a high percentage of the people who diet and lose weight do so only to gain it back within a few years. Why is this? I've found that most depend on a short-term plan or diet to assure long-term success. They planned a two- or three-month program, but again, short-term solutions do not produce long-term results. Those who change their habits by following a realistic eating pattern and exercise program can make changes that last a lifetime.

Maintaining Results

To maintain your results, focus daily on the six steps previously discussed throughout the chapters:

1. **Choose to change from the inside out.** Always remind yourself why you must change and improve the quality of your life. Don't blame anyone or anything—take responsibility and move forward. Our thoughts affect our choices.

2. **Use wisdom.** Follow the facts regarding weight loss, not the fiction.

3. **Choose self-discipline over regret.** The pain of discipline is momentary and rewarding; the pain of regret lingers and is painful.

4. **Prepare ahead.** Planning allows you to prepare, and those who prepare have significantly higher odds of success.

5. **Make the right choices.** Once you make a decision, it then makes you. Focus on the 80/20 rule: Choose correctly in regard to healthy food at least 80 percent of the time. People in special circumstances, such as those on the mission field or on a low income, can't always do this, but God sees your heart and understands your desire to improve your health. Turn it over to Him.

6. **Put first things first.** Prioritizing is placing a majority of your energy on those things that matter and staying the course.

Supplements

Although *What Works When "Diets" Don't* was not written to discuss supplements in detail, a few essential facts need to be included. Supplements can play a key role in weight loss as well as maintaining the results you've worked so hard to achieve. They can be healthy or harmful, depending on the type of supplements you choose.

Stimulants

Stimulants have gained popularity over the years because they temporarily aid weight loss by curbing appetite and speeding up metabolism. But remember, your main goal is health, and stimulants aren't healthy. Caffeine is also a stimulant and, if used, should be used in moderation.

Stimulants have many adverse side effects. Ask yourself, "What is the risk to my health versus the benefit to my health?" Are the benefits going to outweigh the risks? I doubt it! Your heart and organs work very hard, and they don't need the added stress. As an example, some race cars are supercharged to run a quarter-mile in seconds flat, but the engine needs to be replaced, or at least repaired, after every race. The same is true for your body. If you push it beyond where it's designed to go, its performance won't last! Take the safest route, not the fastest. Understand that pills are not the answer. Dinitrophenol was used in the 1930s, rainbow pills in the '60s, amphetamines in the '70s and '80s, fen-phen in the '90s, and massive amounts of caffeine today—none are the answer, and all bring risks. Don't make the same mistake!

Beyond the health risks associated with the use of stimulants (also known as appetite suppressants) is the concern that once the stimulant, or appetite suppressant, is discontinued, your body will crave the calories that were temporarily lacking because of the suppressant. As a result, most people gain the weight back when the stimulants are discontinued. Again, take your time and do it correctly, and weight gain won't be as likely.

Fitness is about health. It's not a race; however, there is a prize: Years added to a healthier life. Align your priorities with your long-term goal. Without health, weight loss seems insignificant!

Supplements are often categorized as follows:

1. Supplements that increase anaerobic (weight training) performance such as creatine or glutamine are popular with fitness enthusiasts. They're primarily used to increase performance and muscle growth and to protect from catabolism (the deterioration of tissue). These supplements aid in building and repairing muscle when taken in moderation.

2. Others, as discussed earlier, enhance energy levels and, in some cases, decrease appetite. Some companies combine caffeine and other harmful stimulants to deliver a more powerful punch. Avoid these supplements, especially in combination.

3. Some supplements are crucial to your success: vitamins and minerals. Although most people are aware of the role vitamins and minerals play in their overall health, they still fail to use them. Many health problems can be linked to a vitamin or mineral deficiency within the body. Proper supplementation (i.e., vitamins and minerals) can provide you with the nutrients needed to protect against deficiencies. When you exercise or eliminate certain foods from your diet, you lose vitamins and minerals. In an attempt to replenish the vitamin and mineral deficit, your body will become hungry, craving nutrients that are lacking. Proper supplementation fights unneeded hunger and weight gain as well as strengthens your immune system! It's also nearly impossible to receive sufficient amounts of vitamins and minerals while monitoring caloric intake; therefore, supplementation is a necessity. Additional supplements that contain ingredients such as organic and non-GMO barley malt, chlorella, alfalfa, grape seed extract, wheatgrass, and bee pollen, for example, are often highly recommended.

For additional information on supplements, see my books *Feasting and Fasting* or *HELP! I'm Addicted.*

Secret to Success

Most of us desire to be in great shape and good health. Unfortunately, desire alone is not enough. Any great feat began with someone's passionate action! For the number of people today who want to get in shape, far too few arrive! Why? We often desire the results without the effort, and we want the reward without earning it.

In the past, a day's work meant plowing the field, cutting firewood, preparing dinner, and organizing the next day's activities. Today, most of us walk forty feet to the car, drive to work, find a parking spot as close to the front door as possible, sit at our desk, and begin work. At the end of the day, we walk to the car, drive home, perhaps purchase an unhealthy dinner on the way, and spend the evening watching the media! Although not true of everyone, it is an indicator of how our society has changed. I'm not suggesting that we return to the past, but it is important to note that this change has created epidemic proportions of obesity and health-related illnesses.

Don't wait until all is going well before you incorporate fitness into your lifestyle—you may wait a lifetime. Start now, regardless of your current situation. Those who succeed walk *through* adversity, not without it! There's no "best" time to start. Begin now, and remember—as long as you take a step forward, even after stepping back, you'll continue to move in the right direction.

If a person desires a good marriage, they need to be a good spouse. If they desire a good job, they need to be a good employee. If they desire a better relationship with their children, they need to be a better parent. In the same way, if you desire to be healthy and fit, apply what it takes to get there.

You are the secret to your success. Despite what you might think, you do have the power to change your life. Research reveals that it's not the circumstances of life that cause failure, but it's our response to them and our attitude that determine success or failure. Success in weight loss truly is 10 percent circumstance and 90 percent attitude.

Where There's Food, There's Life

The Battle Within

There was a young man who decided to visit a local pastor. After years of frustration and regret, he had hit what he considered rock bottom. He needed solid direction for his life. He had worked for several years and had nothing to show for it. He had been easily influenced, and most of his friends were significant contributors to his negative attitude. As a result, his mind was filled with depressing thoughts.

The young man set out to seek advice. He found a pastor busy at work in his study. He told the pastor about his difficult life. He wanted to be a better person, but he couldn't seem to stay on track.

The young man began, "It's almost as if I have two dogs constantly at war within me. One dog is evil and negative, while the other is good and positive!" He continued to say that the battles were very long and challenging; they drained him emotionally and mentally to the point of exhaustion. He explained further that he couldn't seem to make the right choices in life.

Without a moment's thought, the pastor asked the young man, "Which dog wins the battle?" Looking a bit confused, the young man said, "I told you about the constant struggle that leaves me depressed and negative. Isn't it obvious that the evil dog wins?" The pastor looked knowingly at the young man and wisely said, *"Then that's the dog you feed the most! If you want to experience victory, you need to starve that dog to death!"*

Where there's food, there's life...

What we feed grows, and what grows will be the dominating force within our lives. Negativity, anger, resentment, bitterness, and unforgiveness can produce a negative, unproductive attitude! The people we surround ourselves with and the thoughts we entertain will eventually be seen in our actions. Be aware of the thoughts you allow. It's in the mind that success and failure are determined.

Life is a long race, full of wonderful opportunities and experiences.

There are also occasional roadblocks, delays, pitfalls, and hurdles. Make no mistake about it; we win by persevering, by getting up and not giving in. Successful people build success from failure! And they don't look back because it's not the direction they want to go.

Everyone falls, but not everyone gets up! Few things hinder us more than failing to forgive others or ourselves from past mistakes. Many times, they haunt and discourage us from moving forward. As a result, many people rate themselves according to what they were or what they did, not realizing that who they are now and who they will become is far more important.

We live in a world that often will not allow us to forget our past mistakes. There are too few people to encourage or help us along the way. It's sad but true. People will either lift you up or pull you down. If you're not sure if the person is a positive influence, consider where they are leading you. Is it the direction that you want to go?

Like it or not, who we associate with may be who we become! And avoid the "what others say and think" trap. We often judge ourselves by their standards, failing to recognize that what people may say about us is not who we are. Don't let their opinion become your reality. Recognize it, acknowledge it, but don't accept it!

With life comes power. The power to persevere is one of the strongest attributes that we possess. Learning from experience empowers us to move forward. There is little we can do about life's glitches—except control the way we respond to them. Remember that the obstacles ahead are never as high as the power of hindsight.

Getting in Shape Is Not as Hard as It Appears

Society tends to program our looks and actions. Women, as well as young girls, reference magazines to see how they should dress and act. Teenage boys consult the media for role models. And many men today measure their self-worth by what they have accomplished in business and financial matters, not realizing that relationships with family and others are the treasure they should be seeking. What a sad commentary on the state of our society today.

We have become a society focused on prosperity instead of provision, we value money over morals, and we are drawn to charisma instead of character. It's little wonder that our nation's overall health is rapidly declining.

It began inwardly and has spread outwardly. Character qualities like discipline, perseverance, patience, and commitment are almost nonexistent in today's society or have been grossly misused. Failure to adhere to these basic principles has eroded character from our lives like time has eroded the banks of the Colorado River and formed the Grand Canyon. Erosion can occur so slowly that we are unaware of it until its work is done. It has the power to change a river's course. And surely erosion can change the course of our lives. Don't allow a declining cultural mindset to erode the essential qualities we are capable of achieving, such as discipline, perseverance, commitment, determination, and patience. They are essential to the strength and character required to produce lasting results. The true message of this book is simple and straightforward: Your life is merely a reflection of the choices you make. If you are unhappy, simply make other choices.

Conclusion

In closing, losing weight is not as hard as it appears. Establish a goal and stay committed. Control your thoughts, move forward, and ignore setbacks. Prioritize your time, eat clean, move more, fast, and stay motivated. Sound difficult? Not really. Most of us already do these things. We have goals, but sometimes they are the wrong ones. We have time, but we frequently misappropriate it. We have priorities, but they're sometimes misplaced. We feed our thoughts but often with the wrong information. And we're disciplined, but only in certain areas of our lives. For example, the disciplined single parent who works long hours to provide for their family doesn't have to lack discipline when it comes to their health. It's all about choices.

A true measure of a person is not what they were but what they will become!

CHAPTER EIGHT

Step

The Important Discipline of Fasting

(Special excerpt from my book *Feasting and Fasting*)

A s stated earlier, you choose: Will it be the pain of discipline or the pain of regret? One yields a sense of extreme fulfillment; the other, a lingering sense of defeat. Ironically, we pray for God to heal when we should also pray for the self-discipline to change harmful habits. Fasting is hard because self-denial is hard (discipline), and overindulging is not rewarding (regret). It becomes a never-ending cycle of defeat unless we break the cycle by choosing discipline over regret as we seek the will of God.

God teaches us through discipline because He loves us. We are also encouraged to discipline our bodies. We cannot effectively be filled with the Spirit and lack discipline. Our faith is not passive; it's active faith. Romans 6:16 (NASB) sheds much-needed light: "Do you not know that when you present yourselves to someone as slaves for obedience, you are slaves of the one whom you obey, either of sin resulting in death, or of obedience resulting in righteousness?" Either way, we are slaves—we are either God's servant or a slave to our passions and desires. Self-discipline is a fruit of the Spirit, according to 2 Timothy 1:7. Those who say that discipline is legalism are dead wrong. We are called to yield to the Spirit and quench sin—but when we yield to sin, we quench the Spirit. Fleshly appetites are subdued when fasting. Fasting is challenging because the flesh always wants to negotiate with us. It says, "Can't we meet in the middle? Don't completely remove food—that's too extreme!"

Self-control is also required for leadership. In Titus 1:8 (NIV), Paul adds that a leader "must be hospitable, one who loves what is good, who is self-controlled, upright, holy and disciplined." John Wesley required fasting so that his leaders disciplined their appetites rather than allowed their appetites to rule them. It's been said for centuries that no man who cannot command himself is fit to command another. Paul told the Corinthians that he strikes a blow to his body and makes it his slave so that he will not be disqualified for service (1 Cor. 9:27). An undisciplined leader is an oxymoron.

We also see the power of fasting in Joel 1:14: "Consecrate a fast, call a sacred assembly; gather the elders and all the inhabitants of the land into the house of the Lord your God, and cry out to the Lord." The magnitude of the situation determined the response. God's people had departed from Him, not unlike today. The call was to return through fasting, prayer, and brokenness. Fasting is depriving the flesh of its appetite as we pray and seek God's will and mercy. We are saying, "The flesh got me into this predicament, now it's time to seek God's mercy and humble myself before Him."

Obviously, people have overcome challenges without fasting, but fasting adds extra strength, especially when overcoming addictions. Fasting is not a cure-all; it's a spiritual discipline designed to aid in victory. Again, choose the pain of discipline over the pain of regret.

Fasting—The Physical Affects the Spiritual

Through fasting, our body becomes a servant instead of a master. When Jesus directs us, the outcome is always beneficial, spiritually and physically. Notice He said, "When you fast" (Matt. 6:16). Scripture doesn't say, "When you sin, and if you fast," but rather, "If you sin" and "When you fast." The obvious goal and benefit of fasting is spiritual, but there are physical benefits as well. Can we pray and seek God with all our heart with a headache, tight pants, and a sluggish, lethargic body strung out on our favorite addictive substance? Of course not. Does the way you feel affect your productivity and the quality of your life? Absolutely. Our diet affects key hormones such as serotonin for relaxation, dopamine for pleasure, glutamate for healthy thinking, and noradrenaline for handling stress. If we allow junk food and addictions to control our attitude and productivity, it will hinder what we do for God. When we're always dealing with stress, anxiety, and sickness, can we do much for God? No, we will be limited. Granted, there are those who, through no fault of their own, have a debilitating illness. I'm assuming the reader understands that I'm talking to those who can make changes.

What you put in the mouth (body) and the mind (soul) affects the spirit—and when you feed the spirit, it affects the body and the soul. I'm often asked to pray for panic attacks, angry outbursts, and anxiety. That can be done, and God honors prayer, but are we opening the door to these things by not halting highly addictive caffeine, sugar, opioid, or nicotine habits? Or are we renewing our mind by meditating on the Word and spending time in prayer? The physical affects the spiritual, and the spiritual affects the physical. Much of the healing that I have witnessed over the years was the result of renewed stewardship of the body.

We also know that many emotions such as anger, bitterness, and jealousy are toxic to the body. Health also involves healthy emotions. Having a forgiving, loving, joy-filled heart does wonders for the body. Serotonin, for example, is increased when the heart is right. This crucial chemical (also affected by diet and exercise) impacts our mood at a very deep level and contributes to an overall state of well-being.

Again, I'm not suggesting that health should replace God and prayer but that it should complement them—that we steward the gift of health. No one is perfect, but we are called to discipline our bodies and use wisdom. God does heal miraculously, even in our ignorance, but that shouldn't cause us to neglect our health.

With more than 12 million US children being obese, and millions more being malnourished, the need to address this topic has never been greater. Caffeine, soft drinks, and junk food are fueling the disease epidemic. **Yet we pray for God to heal rather than ask for His help with the self-discipline to change harmful habits.** What's wrong with this picture? "There are multitudes of diseases which have their origin in fullness, and might have their end in fasting."[25]

The myth that fasting is bad for you is unfounded and has been disproved numerous times. Be careful when getting counsel from those who profit from that advice or from those who know little about how the body heals itself. I vividly recall the story of a man who had colon surgery yet may not have needed it had he just changed his diet. The hospital even fed him a greasy sloppy joe after he awoke from surgery. A lack of wisdom has been our downfall. (For more about how the physical affects the spiritual, search for "The Doctrine of Man (Sin & the Curse)" at WCFAV.org.)

It's been estimated that nearly 75 percent of US clinical trials in medicine are paid for by private companies who benefit. For example, "Statins are good for you"—paid for by pharmaceutical companies that make them.[26] Or "Take this drug to feel better"—never mind the fact that side effects include internal bleeding, seizures, and panic attacks. Or "Eat this children's cereal"—just ignore the harmful GMOs, food coloring, additives, preservatives, and toxins. America, wake up! You are what you eat. **Fasting doesn't kill us; overconsumption and consuming empty food does.** Companies are often driven by revenue, but no one profits from fasting except the faster. Processed food is cheap and convenient. It often contains stimulating and addictive ingredients and flavor-enhancing chemicals. When was the last time you saw an advertisement for broccoli, blueberries, or kale?

Disease is often a problem of toxicity created by what we consume, ingest, or breathe—and fasting is the detox solution. Granted, spiritual health and wholeness are the goals when fasting, but the physical benefits are worthwhile. Dr. J. H. Tilden said, "After fifty-five years of sojourning in the wilderness of medical therapeutics, I am forced to declare . . . that fasting is the only reliable, specific, therapeutic eliminant known to man."[27]

Dr. Joel Fuhrman noted, "The body's wondrous ability to [self-digest] and destroy needless tissue such as fat, tumors, blood vessel plaque, and other nonessential and diseased tissues, while conserving essential tissues, gives the fast the ability to restore . . . youth to the system."[28] Most research on cancer and fasting supports the healing process as well. For example, the goal of chemotherapy is to stop or slow the growth of cancer cells, but it's been said that the body has a natural, God-given way to do this without harming the healthy cells—fasting. Fasting is not a panacea; it simply provides an environment for healing.

Dr. Yuri Nikolayev, a psychiatrist at the University of Moscow, treated schizophrenics with water fasts for 25 to 30 days. This was followed by eating healthy foods for 30 days. About 70 percent of his patients remained free from symptoms for the duration of the 6-year study. The health benefits of fasting are incredible.[29]

Did you know that Type 2 diabetes is nearly eliminated with proper diet when you stop fueling the disease and fast? It doesn't have to be a progressive disease. There is hope if you starve the fuel source and incorporate fasting. The reason you may find it nearly impossible to fast is because you might be withdrawing from poisons and addictive substances. Therefore, begin by eliminating junk food and educate yourself by reading the recommended resources. Seek medical support and consultation if need be, but keep in mind that most are not supportive of fasting simply because they are trained to ease the pain rather than eliminate the problem.

Drugs often don't cure the underlying problem, and they are toxic. Granted, there may be a time for certain medications, but they should be the last resort, not the first. For example, antibiotics wipe out harmful bacteria as well as good bacteria, and some antibiotics can even be harmful. For instance, check out the side effects on WebMD for Ciprofloxacin (Cipro).[30] It even has black box warnings, the strictest labeling requirements the FDA can mandate for prescription drugs. Not only is it prescribed, it's overprescribed and given to kids and the elderly. Yes, all antibiotics have side effects, but doesn't that tell us something?[31] If the underlying problem of poor health isn't dealt with, illness will return with vengeance. **This is why many are chronically sick—they are always medicating and never healing.**

Fasting also lowers blood pressure and impacts blood sugar levels. If you're taking medication for either, you may find yourself over-medicating because the fast is working in conjunction with the medication, albeit naturally. *Medicine often takes the credit when it was God's design that did the healing.*

Again, fasting does not heal the body; it gives the body the optimal environment for healing. Fasting is a process that God created. Additionally, God-given food promotes life; man-created food does not. A recent example of this involved my youngest daughter. She was not breathing well at night. The physician said that her tonsils and adenoids were inflamed and needed to be removed. Knowing that tonsils and adenoids help with immunity, we tried a different route first. We completely changed her diet by removing all sugar (except light fruit and minimal dark honey). We focused on life-giving food and a daily nap. She was breathing well within a week, and an ear infection that had been lingering healed as well. The right nutrition, along with deep sleep, creates a powerful environment for healing. Are you receiving both?

A few months later, another daughter was advised to take amoxicillin for a tooth infection. The dentist said he would remove the tooth and install a metal brace for her to wear for a year. A quick diet change also resulted in her body healing itself, eliminating the need for any dental intervention. **Again, there may be a time for medication, but it should be the last resort, not the first.**

I have friends who are doctors, and I deeply respect them. They are highly trained in easing symptoms. But most in the healthcare industry are not educated in fixing the cause. For example, many men are told to take AndroGel because of low testosterone levels, but they can often increase their testosterone naturally by avoiding alcohol, exercising, eating healthy food, eliminating sugar, lowering stress, fasting, and taking vitamin D. I knew a man whose testosterone level went from 225 to 530 within eight months by changing his lifestyle. The side effects of testosterone therapy should be motivation enough to make changes.

A few years ago, a doctor wanted to send me home with two different high blood pressure medications. Before leaving, I asked him if he used the large cuff for men when he took my blood pressure. He didn't. When he did, the blood pressure reading came in normal. I can list many more examples of inconsistency, such as a sign in a doctor's office that said in big letters right above the coffee pot: "DON'T CONSUME BEFORE A STRESS TEST." Let's wake up! Our health is on the line.

We need more physicians who understand how the body works and can help the patient from the inside out. They need us, and we need them. But I cringe at the number of Type 2 diabetes patients who are sent home from their doctor's office with even more medication or the countless overweight individuals who leave with high blood pressure drugs instead of real solutions that work. Sadly, we often prefer the "quick fix" approach. But please don't misunderstand—I'm not suggesting that we bypass prayer, nor am I insinuating that we disregard the advice of physicians or that we don't need medication. We must use wisdom. Again, I have seen God heal primarily through fixing the toxic state of the body. How can we pray, "Lord, please heal my heart disease," while driving to McDonald's?

(Again, this chapter was taken from my book *Feasting and Fasting.* At the time of this writing, you can find free downloads at certain retailers and at WCFAV.org.)

A Personal Note from the Author

I want to share with you the most important decision I've ever made. Although I was earning a six-figure income, the years during my late twenties were the worst years of my life. *I was driven, but for the wrong reasons. I felt a sense of purpose, but it left me feeling empty. I was passionate, but for the wrong things.*

I was raised by a loving Christian mother and hard-working father who taught me integrity, honesty, and other qualities, but I never wholeheartedly embraced a personal relationship with God. *I focused on everything the world had to offer, but ultimately, I found that it offered nothing.*

Desperate for direction and fulfillment, I began to search the pages of my Bible shelved long ago with other memorabilia from my past. As I read, two Scriptures seemed to leap from the pages: "For what does it profit a man to gain the whole world, but lose his very soul?" (Luke 9:25) and "When you hear My voice, harden not your heart" (Hebrews 4:7). That was it! I had looked for fulfillment in all the wrong areas. **While I had focused on externals, prosperity, physical fitness, and nutrition, I had *starved* my soul.** I had been independent, self-centered, and prideful. I had hardened my heart against God.

I continued to consume the pages of my Bible, and as a result, I recommitted my life to Christ. Within the months that followed, my passion and my purpose for life became more evident than ever before. And direction? Well, direction was unclear. However, I was now open for wherever His lead might take me.

I would soon walk away from a lucrative career and face the unknown to write this book. It was a time of financial uncertainty but apparent spiritual certainty. Psalms 32:8 helped to ease my mind: "I will instruct you and teach you in the way you should go; I will guide you with My eye." I may not have known where my steps were lead-ing, but God did.

I took a monumental step in writing this section. Many believe that expressing Christian principles and a relationship with God dramatically threatens marketability. **But my focus is no longer on marketability but credibility and responsibility.** I believe people respect the truth and are hungry for it. We are to do what is right, not what is popular.

I hope that you sense within the pages of this book of the great need to apply spiritual principles for success. Committing to these principles helps to assure the completion of a successful weight-loss program. They are sound principles that will help in all areas of life. Although commitment to physical health and fitness has been the dominant theme throughout this book, the most significant commit-ment that you will make is to develop and guard your spiritual health.

If you're searching but not finding, hurting and not healing, and living but not loving, I encourage you to look to the One who has the answers, repent, and commit your life to Him. A true measure of a person is not who they were but who they will become!

A List of Pastor Shane's Other Books

Help! I'm Addicted: Overcoming the Cravings that Overcome You: We are at a crossroads. Opioid and alcohol abuse are leaving a path of destruction in their wake. Pornography is desecrating families. Obesity is skyrocketing and plaguing millions, reaching epidemic levels in children. Heart disease and cancer are—by far—the leading "killers" in America. And on and on it goes, from nicotine to caffeine to food. As a society, we are out of control. But are there answers? Yes, absolutely—if we once again set our sights on God's truth.

Fasting & Feasting: Through fasting, the body becomes a servant instead of a master. The goal and benefit of fasting is spiritual, but the physical benefits as well. Can you pray and seek God better with a headache, tight pants, and a sluggish, lethargic body strung out on your favorite addictive substance? Of course not. But keep in mind that fasting is not about self-reliance but reliance on God

Desperate for More of God: This book is a compilation of past articles, sections from other books I've written, and sermons preached at Westside Christian Fellowship—the best-of-the-best. We pray that this collection of targeted topics fuels an intense desire for more of God. Though the road ahead may be uncertain at times, the solid ground beneath will never shift. It's all about Who you know. Desperate for More should be the heart cry of every believer.

Answers for a Confused Church: There is a dangerous trend in the evangelical church today. A futile attempt is being made to conform God's Word to social norms, rather than to conform social norms to His Word. As a result, truth is vague, doctrine is blurred, and the fundamentals of the Christian faith are often avoided. For this reason, this book outlines some key issues confronting the church today such as absolute truth, unity, judging, abortion, sexual sin, politics, compromise, revival, preaching, repentance, and so on.

One Nation "Above" God: America is divided on many fronts. Where are the answers? How will the future and security of America unfold in the days to come? My previous books address personal issues. This book, however, recognizes the biblical foundation that once guided America. These principles are the foundation on which America's success rests.

What Works for Young Adults: What are the top questions on the minds of young adults today? This question was presented nationally to church and youth leaders, and to young adults themselves— if they have ever needed solid answers, it's now. With practicality, What Works for Young Adults provides fresh answers to provoking questions.

What Works for Men: A down to earth, practical and doable guide to becoming a man of character. Today's cultural norms often run contrary to principles designed to promote healthy masculinity. In a bold approach, the author challenges cultural views and directs the reader back to sound principles.

What Works for Singles: This is a motivational, biblically based resource for those divorced, those marrying for the first time, and those currently single. In all cases, readers will be given the information they need to experience lasting fulfillment.

Notes

1   "The U.S. Weight Loss & Diet Control Market," ResearchandMarkets.com, February 2019, https://www.researchandmarkets.com/research/qm2gts/the_72_billion?w=4.

2   Boston Medical Center, "Weight Management," accessed December 30, 2019, https://www.bmc.org/nutrition-and-weight-management/weight-management.

3   Statista Research Department, "What are your 2018 resolutions?" Statista, August 9, 2019, https://www.statista.com/statistics/378105/new-years-resolution.

4   University of California San Francisco, "How Much Is Too Much?" SugarScience, https://sugarscience.ucsf.edu/the-growing-concern-of-overconsumption.html#.XgqPiEd-KiUl.

5   Alexander Kunst, "Frequency of soft drink consumption worldwide 2017, by country" Statista, December 20, 2019, https://www.statista.com/statistics/695690/frequency-of-soft-drink-consumption-by-country.

6   National Research Council (US); Institute of Medicine (US); Woolf SH, Aron L, editors, "U.S. Health in International Perspective: Shorter Lives, Poorer Health," accessed December 30, 2019, https://www.ncbi.nlm.nih.gov/books/NBK154469.

7   Stuart Wolpert, "Dieting does not work, UCLA researchers report," April 3, 2007, UCLA Newsroom, http://newsroom.ucla.edu/releases/Dieting-Does-Not-Work-UCLA-Researchers-7832.

8   "Chronic Diseases in America," CDC.gov, accessed December 30, 2019, https://www.cdc.gov/chronicdisease/resources/infographic/chronic-diseases.htm.

9   Sara Police, "How Much Have Obesity Rates Risen Since 1950?" Livestrong.com, accessed December 30, 2019, https://www.livestrong.com/article/384722-how-much-have-obesity-rates-risen-since-1950/.

10   "Type 2 Diabetes Statistics and Facts," Healthline, accessed December 30, 2019, https://www.healthline.com/health/type-2-diabetes/statistics.

11   "What are the leading causes of death in the US?" Medical News Today, accessed December 30, 2019, https://www.medicalnewstoday.com/articles/282929.php.

12   "1 in 2 people will develop cancer in their lifetime," Medical News Today, accessed December 30, 2019, https://www.medicalnewstoday.com/articles/288916.php#1.

13   Melonie Heron, Ph.D, "Deaths: Leading Causes for 2017," June 24, 2019, National Vital Statistics Reports, https://www.cdc.gov/nchs/data/nvsr/nvsr68/nvsr68_06-508.pdf.

14   ASN Staff, "Millions of cardiovascular deaths attributed to not eating enough fruits and vegetables," American Society for Nutrition, June 8, 2019, https://nutrition.org/millions-of-cardiovascular-deaths-attributed-to-not-eating-enough-fruits-and-vegetables.

15   Jamie Ducharme, "About 90% of Americans Don't Eat Enough Fruits and Vegetables," Time, November 17, 2017, https://time.com/5029164/fruit-vegetable-diet.

16   Peggy Peck, "Cause of Most Heart Attacks Found," WebMD, accessed December 30, 2019, https://www.webmd.com/heart-disease/news/20040830/cause-of-most-heart-at-tacks-found.

17   "GMO Facts," Non GMO Project, accessed December 30, 2019, https://www.nongmo-project.org/gmo-facts.

18   "The Truth About Aspartame Side Effects," accessed December 31, 2019, Healthline, https://www.healthline.com/health/aspartame-side-effects.

19   "Dirty Dozen™ EWG's 2019 Shopper's Guide to Pesticides in Produce," Environmental Working Group, accessed December 31, 2019, https://www.ewg.org/foodnews/dirty-doz-en.php.

20   "Clean Fifteen™ EWG's 2019 Shopper's Guide to Pesticides in Produce," Environmental Working Group, accessed December 31, 2019, https://www.ewg.org/foodnews/clean-fif-teen.php.

21   Answers in Genesis provides a well-documented chart entitled "Timeline for the Flood" at https://answersingenesis.org/bible-timeline/timeline-for-the-flood.

22   JA Levine, "Non-exercise activity thermogenesis (NEAT)," PubMed.gov, December 16, 2002, https://www.ncbi.nlm.nih.gov/pubmed/12468415.

23   Pedro A. Villablanca MD, et al., "Nonexercise Activity Thermogenesis in Obesity Man-agement," Mayo Clinic, April 2015, https://doi.org/10.1016/j.mayocp.2015.02.001.

24   Dr. Daniel Pompa, "The Truth about Diet Restriction and Weight Loss," May 21, 2019, https://drpompa.com/fasting-diet/ttruth-diet-restriction-weight-loss.

25   James Morrison, quoted in Arthur Wallis, God's Chosen Fast (Fort Washington, PA: Christian Literature Crusade, 1977), 104–105 (emphasis added).

26   See "New Cholesterol Guidelines May Put 13 Million More on Statin Drugs" at Merco-la.com, https://articles.mercola.com/sites/articles/archive/2014/04/02/cholesterol-sta-tin-drugs-guidelines.aspx.

27   Dr. J. H. Tilden, quoted in Herbert M. Shelton, Fasting Can Save Your Life (Tampa: Natural Hygiene Press, 1981), 36. Although I don't agree with all of Dr. Tilden's views, state-ments like this are very common in his books and articles regarding preventative health-care.

28   Joel Fuhrman, Fasting and Eating for Health: A Medical Doctor's Program for Con-quering Disease (New York: St. Martin's Griffin, 1995).

29   Dr. Yuri Nikolayev's research was conducted as the director of the fasting treatment unit of Moscow Psychiatric Institute.

30   See https://www.webmd.com/drugs/2/drug-1124-93/cipro-oral/ciprofloxacin-oral/details.

31   The US National Library of Medicine National Institutes of Health released an article outlining some of the side effects here: https://www.ncbi.nlm.nih.gov/pmc/articles/ PMC3421593, or search online for "Adverse Effects of Antimicrobials via Predictable or Idiosyncratic Inhibition of Host Mitochondrial Components."

Made in the USA
Las Vegas, NV
12 June 2022

50120935R00080